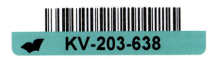

The

Therapy of Pain

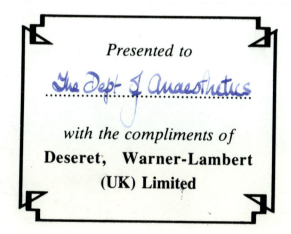

To my wife
Elizabeth Swerdlow

The
Therapy of Pain

Edited by
Mark Swerdlow

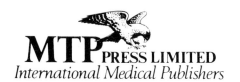

MTP PRESS LIMITED
International Medical Publishers

Published by
MTP Press Limited
Falcon House
Lancaster, England

Copyright © 1981 MTP Press Limited

First published 1981

British Library Cataloguing in Publication Data

The Therapy of Pain (Current status of modern therapy; vol. 6)
I. Pain
I. Swerdlow, Mark   II. Series
616'.047   RB127

ISBN 0-85200-259-9

Typeset by Swiftpages Ltd., Liverpool
Printed in Great Britain by Butler and Tanner Ltd., Frome and London

Contents

List of Contributors

ALLAN S. BROWN
Department of Surgical Neurology, Western General Hospital, Crewe Road, Edinburgh EH4 2XV, Scotland

EDWARD HITCHCOCK
Professor of Neurosurgery and Neurology, Holly Lane, Smethwick, Warley, West Midlands B67 7JX, England

ROBERT D. HUNTER
Consultant Radiotherapist, Christie Hospital and Holt Radium Institute, Withington, Manchester M20 4BX, England

SAMPSON LIPTON
Centre for Pain Relief, Department of Medical and Surgical Neurology, Walton Hospital, Liverpool L9 1AE, England

MARK MEHTA
Pain Relief Service, United Norwich Hospitals, Norwich NR1 3SR, England

ISSY PILOWSKY
Professor of Psychiatry, Department of Psychiatry, University of Adelaide, GPO Box 498, Adelaide, South Australia 5000

DAME CICELY SAUNDERS
Medical Director, St Christopher's Hospice, 51 Lawrie Park Road, Sydenham, Kent SE26 6DZ, England

WILLIAM H. SWEET
Harvard Medical School, Massachusetts General Hospital, One Longfellow Place, Suite 201, Boston, MA 02114, USA

MARK SWERDLOW
Consultant, Regional Pain Relief Centre, Hope Hospital, University of Manchester School of Medicine, Eccles Old Road, Salford M6 8HD, England

NORTON E. WILLIAMS
Consultant Anaesthetist, Whiston Hospital, Prescot, Merseyside L35 5DR, England

BARRY D. WYKE
Director, Neurological Unit, The Royal College of Surgeons of England, 35 Lincoln's Inn Fields, London WC2A 3PN, England

Consultant Editor's Note

Current Status of Modern Therapy

Series Editor: J. Marks, Girton College, Cambridge

The *Current Status of Modern Therapy* is a major new series from MTP Press with the purpose of providing a definitive view of modern therapeutic practice in those areas of clinical medicine in which important changes are occurring. The series consists of monographs specially commissioned under the individual editorship of internationally recognized experts in their fields. Their selection of a panel of contributors from many countries ensures an international perspective on developments in therapy.

The series will aim to review the growth areas of clinical pharmacology and therapeutics in a systematic way. It will be a continuing series in which the same subject areas will be covered by revised editions as advances make this desirable.

Pain is a symptom of disorder within the body and is one of the most unpleasant emotional experiences known to humans. This applies whatever the underlying cause. Hence effective appropriate therapy is vitally important.

The major development over the past few decades has been the establishment of specialized 'Pain Clinics' with a multidisciplinary approach and Mark Swerdlow was one of the pioneers in the area. For this volume he has collected a group of experts in their respective fields. Each has taken an eminently practical approach in the chapter he has written. In consequence this is a worthy volume for the series.

Preface

The past few years have seen the publication of a large number of articles and not a few books on the subject of relief of intractable pain. New ideas have been put forward on pain mechanisms, new methods of treatment have been reported and improved results claimed, and a growing catalogue of complications of treatment has been recorded. The vast and expanding literature on the subject poses for the reader the dual problems of surveillance and of assessment. The object of the present book is to provide a critical and constructive review of current writings and ideas on a wide range of aspects of the nature of intractable pain, particularly of present day practice and new ideas on treatment. Each chapter is written by an acknowledged authority and the approach throughout is practical rather than academic. In editing the individual chapters an effort was made to achieve a contemporary approach and to eliminate material which was unduly historical or retrospective in content. At the same time the individual style of the authors was retained as far as possible.

For decades chronic pain has been a therapeutic 'no man's land'. For the surgeon pain was an unfortunate complication which not infrequently followed surgery; for the physician it was a distressing symptom in a number of disease syndromes; to the psychiatrist it was one of a number of features in many cases of mental illness. To the doctor who works in a pain relief clinic, however, the study and treatment of pain are his 'raison d'être'.

The earliest 'Pain Clinics' were set up in the 1940s and were essentially nerve block clinics. In the late 1960s the importance of a multidisciplinary approach became recognized. In particular, close inter-speciality discussion and consultation counteract the almost inevitable 'tunnel vision' approach of each individual specialist. The past decade or more has seen an increasing number of pain relief centres established in many countries. The way in which these clinics function, the kind and number of specialities involved and the degree of integration show marked differences. The chapter on 'Current Views on the Management of a Pain Relief Centre' looks at the different ways of achieving an efficient unit and provides valuable comments and advice. It will be found useful by those about to set up a clinic and thought-provoking by those already established in pain centres. However it is written in the context of the British Health Service and readers in other countries may have to make modifications to suit their own medical service conditions.

Advances in our knowledge of the neurophysiology of pain have been at the spearhead of many of the recent advances in pain therapy. The chapter on neurophysiology provides a broad review of our current knowledge of this field, with all its practical significance and applications, including much information on the natural chemical transmitter substances. There is a steady development of new drugs of value to patients suffering from chronic pain and the number and types of drug employed are changing so rapidly that the pharmacology textbooks cannot keep pace and fail to provide information on many newer therapeutic practices. The chapter on pharmacology will be found to give an up-to-date, balanced account of the current value and usage of a wide variety of drugs in pain therapy.

Pain caused by cancer is one of the most distressing and demoralizing forms of human suffering and is a great challenge to the staff of the pain relief clinic. Methods of relieving cancer pain are discussed in a number of chapters, particularly in Chapters 8 and 9, which deal respectively with the role of the oncologist and with pain relief in terminal care. The reader will also find some interesting views on the developing relationship between pain clinics and terminal care units.

In other chapters present day opinions on the place and value of proper psychological management are reviewed and discussed, as are conventional methods such as nerve blocks, neurosurgery etc., which may be necessary to deal with one or other of the many conditions causing pain. The chapter on 'Non-invasive Methods' includes a number of procedures and techniques, namely vibrator therapy, ultrasonics, lasers and trigger points, which can on occasion be of value and which have as yet received relatively little reporting.

Preface

There is little doubt that the spread and growth of the 'pain clinic movement' will continue, as medically 'advanced' countries augment the
number and quality of such clinics and countries at present without these
facilities endeavour to introduce them as they become aware of their value.
The fact that theoretical and practical courses are available in many
countries for those with an interest in the subject should ensure the supply
of physicians for future pain relief teams. However the dedicated future
pain workers will probably not come entirely from anaesthesiological
nerve block clinics nor from psychiatrists interested in psychosomatic pain
problems. It is likely that many will have worked in active multidisciplinary centres and will have seen the results that can be achieved, as well as the
fascinating and rewarding research which can be undertaken to investigate
the problems which pain sets. Certainly they will need to have empathy for
people as well as having scientific knowledge.

It is hoped that this book will be useful for neurosurgeons, psychiatrists,
neurologists, anaesthetists and others who work in pain relief clinics, as
well as for the family doctors and specialists who refer patients to these
clinics.

I would like to thank the Publishers for their co-operation at every stage
of the preparation of this book and especially in the very speedy printing
which was essential if the 'Current Views' were not to become out-of-date
before reaching the reader. I would also like to express my appreciation to
Mrs. Angela Hinks for considerable secretarial help.

MARK SWERDLOW

Foreword

The past 10 years have seen major thrusts: 1 to improve the management of chronic pain; 2 to bring the better methods into more widespread use, and 3 to increase our knowledge of the mechanisms of acute and chronic pain so that further improvements can be guided more intelligently. The achievement of all three of these objectives has been aided by the formation of national societies all over the world. This concept was first widely endorsed at an International Symposium on Pain in Seattle, Washington in May 1973 and the International Association for the Study of Pain (IASP) was formed to coordinate and expand these efforts. The need for such formal organization has been substantiated by the huge attendance at the two World Congresses on 'Pain' which have since been sponsored by IASP.

I must confess that when I learned that national and international societies were being formed confining their purview to the subject of pain, I emitted groans of profound psychological anguish. Already a member of innumerable societies covering a broad range of basic science and clinical disciplines, I thought the formation of a society to deal with a clinical symptom was a move in the wrong direction – at a time when the number of specialized learned societies had already reached revolting proportions. I have lived to change my mind, to be surprised and delighted at the number of intellectual approaches to the problem of pain and the validity of an effort to bring their advocates into intercommunication. Now, within the confines of the individual human effort, there can be a reasonable grasp of the entire field. Now one need not himself be a member of those societies whose discipline makes a contribution to the subject of pain, because all of these disciplines are represented in IASP.

Likewise the published material is happily being concentrated in such journals as *Pain* whose parent association is IASP, and in a number of books. These include the three volumes *Advances in Pain Research and Therapy*, which in Volumes 1 and 3 summarize the proceedings respectively of the first and second World Congresses on Pain. These books must however be classified as relatively non-critical compendia of what various workers did and thought. They are for the specialist in pain, who must himself supply the evaluation of the merit of the many contributions they contain. One must acknowledge that in some quarters there has been more enthusiasm than can be justified by any available thoughtful appraisals.

The need for a comprehensive critique of the field is met by such a book as this one edited by Dr Swerdlow. British physicians have long had a reputation for being able to distinguish between the wheat and the chaff, and the chapters I have been given the opportunity to review in advance uphold this reputation. This book has as well another more major role, namely *it provides the general physician with a readable rundown on the main modes of clinical management of pain at the present time.*

As to the individual chapters in the book I shall comment on only a few. An overview of the greatly expanded role of the psychiatrist and the psychologist is admirably described and documented by Pilowsky. Early in my career my attitude was that I should not hire a psychiatrist to become acquainted with my patient as a person; that was an essential part of *my* job. However I soon had to concede that a skilled psychiatrist who is really interested in patients with chronic pain could do a better job than I of ferreting out the personal and interpersonal problems of the patients. My colleague and co-author for decades, Dr James C. White and I have long recognized the value of these collaborators in the attack on chronic pain. The sceptic will find out from Pilowsky just what the behavioural, psychological and psychiatric approaches to the person disabled by pain have achieved. This essayist selects for citation those articles presenting the long-term followups, crucial to any valid decision as to the place of the methods.

The concepts as well as the administrative and technical details involved in setting up specialized units to deal with pain have been set forth by Lipton, based on his broad experience at the Walton Hospital in Liverpool. I can assure the reader that the advice presented is based on enough success to make it worth heeding. The notion of a multidisciplinary pain clinic is not brand new. That certainly is what René Leriche ran in

Strasbourg in the twenties and thirties and my former chief James C. White set up in the thirties following the examples of Leriche, Foerster and Wertheimer. White, in particular, saw to it that the full intellectual and physical resources of the Massachusetts General Hospital were called into play in patients with persistent pain who came under his care from many parts of the country. However I think the notion is new that if the physician and his colleagues in a general hospital interested in the problem of chronic pain cannot help a patient, they have an obligation to identify or if necessary to help create other facilities manned by other experts who might successfully work with the patient. This in the USA is likely to entail referral of the patient to a chronic care service. All the necessary diagnostic exercises will have been performed in the general hospital, and the 4–8 week re-education which may be required to teach the patient to manage his pain can be more effectively and less expensively spent in a rehabilitation hospital with a group of patients having similar problems. I agree with Lipton that one must not overdo the use of consultants or consultant groups in diagnosing and managing patients with pain. I confess that I disagree with one (but only one) statement of Lipton. He says the use of acupuncture in pain relief is acknowledged. If by acupuncture he means the placement of needles at very precise points in accordance with the prescriptions of Ancient Chinese medical lore, then I know of no controlled study which defines the types of organic pain syndrome in which such manoeuvres are of value.

I add my eager confirmation of one of Dr Hunter's statements in his chapter on oncological methods of pain relief. He emphasizes that unremitting pain may not only be a late manifestation of cancer, it may also be its earliest symptom. On at least five occasions in my experience a relentless, torturing pain, destroying the patient's morale was present for weeks before repeated clinical as well as non-invasive and invasive examinations finally led to proof that it was due to cancer. Previous physicians in charge of each patient had failed to recognize that the disabling intensity of pain carried with it the high index of suspicion that a malignant tumour was at the root of the problem. Intimating to such a patient that he must be exaggerating the magnitude of his discomfort is an excellent way to make him a permanent enemy when the unattractive truth eventually emerges.

I cannot forbear remarking that the neurosurgical management of the pain of advancing cancer may represent a most rewarding experience for the patient and for his physicians. This was brought home to me early in my career when I was the neurosurgeon at the Queen Elizabeth Hospital in

Birmingham during World War II. I performed a technically successful antero-lateral cordotomy on a young man with cancer, relieving his pain. Doing well in his first post-operative week, he abruptly declined and died during the next week. I apologized to the patient's siblings for having submitted their brother to a major operation, which I should not have done had I known death was imminent. With one voice they assured me that they were all most grateful that the operation had been done, that the post-operative period had been the only pain-free days he had had for over a year. In the previous months he had either been in a medicated lethargy or in agony. Their sole regret was that the operation had not been done sooner, and they gave me the first attractive gift I had received from a patient.

I do not criticize the neurosurgeons of the United Kingdom directly for their relative inattention to cancer patients. With only 90 consultant neurosurgeons in the nation they are proportionately a much tinier band of such specialists than are to be found in any other Western European or English-speaking nation. With a few exceptions they are too swamped with other tasks to be able in many centres to attend the patient with advancing cancer. Hence they do not draw to the attention of their other medical colleagues the full extent of the neurosurgical resources for these patients. In the final paragraphs of his chapter Dr Hunter under the rubric 'Clinical Problem Areas', describes five groups of patients in whom 'improved radiotherapeutic, chemotherapeutic, surgical and hormone therapy have failed to make any significant impact and in whom chronic pain is a major problem'. For these patients making small lesions in the white matter of the frontal lobes may relieve not only the focal pains of the organic lesions but the psychological suffering and distress as well. The price in terms of deficit of cognitive and or emotional behaviour is usually negligible and may be imperceptible. Particularly convincing evidence for this statement has been provided by Teuber, Corkin and Twitchell (1976). Hitchcock (1977) and Sweet (1980) have already emphasized the need for wider use of these well established procedures. I commend to the reader especially Hitchcock's chapter since it may well fill a wide gap in his knowledge, and lead to a much wider realization of what neurosurgery has to offer.

References

Hitchcock, E. R. (1977). Small frontal lesions for intractable pain. *Prog. Neurol. Surg.* **8,** 114

Foreword

Sweet, W. H. (1980). Central mechanisms of chronic pain. *Proc. Assoc. Res. Nerv. Ment. Dis.*, **58**, 287

Teuber, H. L., Corkin, S. and Twitchell, T. E. (1977). Appendix #3 to Report of National Commission for the Protection of Human Subjects of Biomedical and Behavioral Research. U.S. Dept. Health, Education and Welfare Publication No. (OS)77–0002, pp. 1–115, 1977. Summarized as 'Study of cingulotomy in man' in *Neurosurgical Treatment in Psychiatry, Pain and Epilepsy*, edited by W. Sweet, S. Obrador and J. G. Martin-Rodriguez, pp. 355–362. (Baltimore: University Park Press)

W. H. SWEET
Harvard Medical School
Boston
Massachussets

1

Neurological aspects of pain therapy
A Review of Some Current Concepts

B. D. Wyke

After a long period of relative inactivity, pain research has exploded in the last twenty years to become the most rapidly developing of all areas of contemporary neurological investigation. Since the swiftly emerging results of this world-wide activity have had (and will continue to have) profound implications for the clinical management of patients in pain, this introductory chapter reviews some of the general principles that have emerged thus far from this hive of investigation as a prelude to the consideration of the various specialized aspects of pain therapy that is presented in the chapters that follow.

THE NATURE OF THE EXPERIENCE OF PAIN

Perhaps the most fundamental change that has taken place in the understanding of pain as a clinical symptom – and one that is particularly germane to consideration of any form of pain therapy – is the belated recognition that pain is not a sensation (as has long been thought, and taught), but is instead an unpleasant emotional experience*. That is to say, pain (although being in all its manifestations a neurological disorder), does not belong to the same category of primary perceptual experiences as do vision, hearing, smell, touch and kinaesthesis (for example), but instead is

---

*This fact was, however, first realized in the 17th century by the Dutch philosopher Benedictus de Spinoza (1632–1677), who (with remarkable prescience) classified pain as 'a localised form of sorrow' – and thus as one of the primary emotions.

an abnormal affective state that is generated in the synaptic systems of some of the same limbic regions of the cerebral cortex (*vid. inf.*) as are all other affective (i.e. emotional) states.

Several important clinical consequences derive from the realization that pain is an unpleasant emotional state and not a primary perceptual experience. The first is that pain is always a symptom and never a physical sign; and hence in dealing with patients in pain (and when assessing the efficacy of its treatment) one is entirely dependent upon the patient's report of his own introspective experience – for only the patient knows whether he is in pain, and how bad is his pain. The so-called 'physical signs' of pain – such as changes in facial expression, muscle tone and posture, in heart rate and arterial blood pressure, in respiratory activity and in gastrointestinal function for instance – are merely reflexogenic concomitants (*q.v.*) of painful experiences, and their magnitude has no necessary quantitative relationship to the intensity of the patient's suffering. Second, precisely because pain is an emotional state it cannot be summoned up *de novo* by any effort of imaginative will (any more than any other emotional state can be) and hence there is no such thing as 'imaginary pain' – even though doctors may sometimes prefer to dismiss their patients' complaints in this way by saying to themselves that 'it is all in the patient's mind'. Third, the traditional belief that pain is a 'sensation' has led to a widespread clinical misapprehension (which has proved unfortunate for many patients) that its intensity must bear a direct quantitative relationship to the intensity of the tissue disturbance that is provoking it, in the same way as the intensity of primary perceptual experiences is related to the intensity of the evocative stimulus: but in fact (as most clinicians experienced in the management of pain come to appreciate sooner or later), there is no necessary correlation between the intensity of the emotional experience that is pain and the degree of tissue abnormality that is evoking it – for reasons that will become apparent later in this chapter.

A further clinical misapprehension that has arisen from this last misguided belief (namely, that pain is a 'sensation') is the view that measurement of a patient's 'pain threshold' provides a guide to the intensity of the suffering he is likely to experience (or is experiencing) when afflicted with a pain-producing lesion somewhere in his body. Unfortunately – and in spite of the considerable time and effort that has been expended over many years in making such measurements in a wide variety of circumstances – determination of an individual's pain threshold has little practical relevance to the clinical problems presented by the diagnosis and treatment of his pain, for the reason that people do not seek medical assistance simply because their pain threshold has been exceeded by some nociceptive stimulus (which situation occurs almost daily in the experience of most people). On the contrary, what brings patients to their doctors to seek relief are situations in which the limits of their 'pain tolerance' have been reached, and this latter parameter of painful experience is highly variable as between different individuals (being influenced, *inter alia*, by age, sex, race and cultural background) and from time to time in any one individual – in contrast to the relative constancy of pain thresholds in the population at large. For these reasons, what is required in a clinical context – particularly in relation to realistic assessment of the effects of various forms of pain therapy – are not measurements of pain threshold but determinations of pain tolerance; and it is in terms of their effectiveness in elevating pain tolerance that therapeutic methods (other than those that result in removal of the primary cause of the pain) should primarily be judged.

In the light of the foregoing observations, then, the present view of the nature of pain may be summarized by saying that it is an emotional disturbance generated in the synaptic systems of certain of the limbic sectors of the cerebral cortex by the arrival therein of impulses of sufficient frequency through specific afferent pathways that constitute the nociceptive system – the term 'nociceptive' signifying 'responding to tissue abnormality'. Since activation of this normally quiescent nociceptive afferent system is the essential prerequisite for the evocation of the experience of pain, some of the clinically relevant features of the peripheral and central components of this afferent system will now be reviewed.

PERIPHERAL NOCICEPTIVE SYSTEMS

Nociceptive receptor systems

Since pain is not a sensation, there are no pain sensory receptors in any tissue in the sense that there are receptor nerve endings anywhere whose stimulation will inevitably evoke the experience of pain and whose frequency of discharge is the primary determinant of the intensity of that experience. But there are morphologically distinct nerve endings in tissues whose activation by various forms of tissue abnormality (*vid. inf.*) may or may not give rise to the experience of pain of varying intensity, depending upon the prevailing activity of a number of modulating influences that operate upon centripetal transmission of activity derived therefrom to the cerebral cortex that will be described later. These nerve endings constitute the nociceptive receptor system – of which there are two varieties in most tissues.

Interstitial nociceptive receptors

In most human tissues (such as skin, adipose tissue, fasciae, periosteum, joint capsules, pleura, pericardium, peritoneum, dura mater and mucous membranes) one type of nociceptive receptor system is represented, not by free nerve endings (which are largely confined to the cornea, the teeth, tendons and the ligaments of joints), but by a continuous tridimensional plexus of unmyelinated nerve fibres that weaves (like chicken-wire) in all directions throughout the tissue.

This plexiform receptor system is normally inactive, but it is provoked into activity when its constituent nerve fibres are depolarized by their exposure to sufficiently severe degrees of mechanical distortion of the tissue in which they are embedded, or to sufficiently marked alterations in the chemical composition of the tissue fluid that bathes them (*q.v.*). In these circumstances, the resulting nociceptive receptor activity is propagated centripetally into the neuraxis through small diameter afferent nerve fibres (*vid. inf.*) that leave the network at its nodes and join the related peripheral nerves.

Perivascular nociceptive receptors

The walls of all arteries, arterioles, venules and veins (but not capillaries) – except those in the brain and spinal cord – likewise contain a similar plexus of unmyelinated nerve fibres that encircles each blood vessel, embedded in its adventitial sheath. Like the interstitial system, this perivascular nociceptive receptor system is stimulated by its mechanical distortion or by its exposure to similar changes in the chemical composition of the surrounding tissue fluid as irritate the interstitial receptor system.

From the above considerations, then, it will be apparent that two important initial questions need to be answered in the differential diagnosis of pain experienced in any part of the body – for upon the answers to such questions will depend (*inter alia*) the rational planning of treatment of the pain in question. The first is, is the pain of mechanical or of chemical origin (or a combination of the two); and the second, is it of interstitial or perivascular origin (or a combination of both). Determination of the answers to these two crucial questions is aided by paying careful attention to the precise qualifying adjectives chosen by a patient when replying to the question 'what is the pain like?' Should the patient choose adjectives that are exclusively descriptive of mechanical experience (such as 'pressing', 'bursting' or 'stabbing', for example) then the pain probably arises from mechanical changes in the tissues; whereas if he chooses the adjective 'burning' he is describing a pain that is chemically provoked. Furthermore, should he choose any mechanical adjective other than 'throbbing', his pain is being provoked by mechanical irritation of the interstitial nociceptive receptor system: but should he select this latter adjective, his pain clearly is of perivascular origin (either mechanical or chemical).

Activation of nociceptive receptor systems
As pointed out above, both the interstitial and perivascular nociceptive receptor systems may be stimulated by sufficiently severe mechanical or chemical abnormalities developing in the various tissues of the body.

Mechanical irritation of interstitial nociceptive receptors is provoked when the tissues containing them are disrupted by their incision, tearing or laceration, or when abnormally high mechanical stresses are generated in the tissues by their excessive stretching or compression. In the case of the perivascular receptor system similar considerations apply, but it should be pointed out that this latter system may be mechanically irritated equally by marked constriction or dilatation of the blood vessels (whether arteries or veins), since it is not the direction but the magnitude of the change in vascular diameter that is the relevant criterion in this case.

Chemical irritation of both interstitial and perivascular nociceptive receptor systems arises when sufficiently high concentrations of a variety of chemical agents accumulate in the surrounding tissue fluid – and the principal substances in this respect are lactic acid, K^+ ions, a variety of polypeptide kinins, 5-hydroxytryptamine, prostaglandin E and histamine. Since lactic acid and K^+ ions are released in high concentrations by the cells of ischaemic tissues, it is hardly surprising that such tissues (and especially muscles) may become painful; and since the other substances are released by traumatized cells, and are also major constituents of inflammatory exudates, it is clear that a chemical component (as well as a mechanical one) contributes to the pain of traumatized tissues and that the pain associated with inflammatory lesions is largely of chemical origin (unless abscess formation occurs, in which case a mechanical element is added as a result of the stretching of the tissues surrounding the abscess).

Peripheral nociceptive afferent systems

All nociceptive afferent fibres in human peripheral nerves (whether of somatic or visceral origin) are less than $5\,\mu$m in diameter – those between $2\,\mu$m and $5\,\mu$m being small myelinated fibres; and those less than $2\,\mu$m in diameter (which are the majority) being unmyelinated. The peripheral nociceptive afferents therefore constitute the smallest diameter afferent system in the body; and upon this fact depends their extemely slow conduction velocity, their very high threshold to electrical excitation, their considerable resistance to ischaemic blockade and their special differential sensitivity to the action of local anaesthetic agents – all matters of considerable clinical importance.

For example, the high resistance of nociceptive afferents to ischaemic blockade is the reason why ischaemic tissues remain painful even though all other modalities of sensation in the tissue (and in the case of the striated muscles their motor control) may have been lost. Again, the special sensitivity of these afferents to relatively low concentrations of local anaesthetic agents provides the means whereby differential analgesia may be produced by injection of appropriate concentrations of such agents (as is possible in the performance of brachial plexus or epidural blocks, for instance). Finally (and especially in relation to matters that will be mentioned later in this chapter and in other chapters of this book), the fact that nociceptive afferents in peripheral nerves have a much higher threshold to electric excitation than do the mechanoreceptor afferents (or somatic motor efferents) in the same nerves underlies the effectiveness of the use of transcutaneous nerve stimulators for the relief of many varieties of pain.

Peripheral modulation of pain

It has already been pointed out that mechanical or chemical irritation of the tissue nociceptive receptor systems that have been described may or may not give rise to the experience of pain, and that even if it does the intensity of the experience is not necessarily a direct function of the intensity of such receptor irritation. This divorce between the intensity of nociceptive receptor stimulation and the intensity of the associated pain (if any) is imposed by the influence of a number of modulating neurological mechanisms operating on the centripetal propagation of nociceptive afferent activity at various synapses within the neuraxis through which such activity is relayed on its way to the cerebral cortex. One such modulating influence is exercised from peripheral tissue mechanoreceptors – and since this peripheral modulating mechanism has proved in recent years to be of considerable clinical importance in the relief of pain, its basic principles are considered here* as a background to the more detailed information in this respect that is provided in later chapters of this book.

In the peripheral nerves distal to the dorsal root ganglia, the nociceptive afferent nerve fibres (Figure 1) are randomly intermingled with the other fibres (afferent and efferent) in such nerves: but as the preganglionic portion of each dorsal root approaches the spinal cord its constituent fibres

---

*In the interests of brevity, this discussion is confined to modulation of pain arising from spinally innervated tissues. Similar principles apply to orofacial pain (although some of the details are necessarily different): a full discussion of the subject of orofacial pain may be found in Wyke (1976) and Anderson and Matthews (1976).

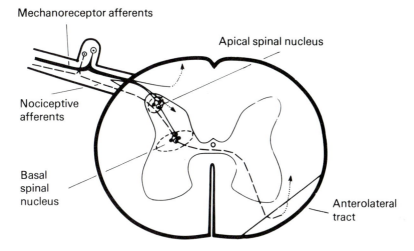

Mechanoreceptor afferents

Apical spinal nucleus

Nociceptive
afferents

Basal
spinal
nucleus

Anterolateral
tract

Figure 1 Diagram illustrating the principles of intraspinal modulation of nociceptive inputs by mechanoreceptor afferents. Description in text

become segregated into two rami in terms of their diameters – all those larger than 5 μm (that is, those innervating the various types of corpuscular mechanoreceptor that are distributed through the peripheral tissues) being diverted into the posterior ramus and those less than 5 μm in diameter (and thus all the nociceptor afferents) into the anterior ramus. As the anteriorly-located nociceptive afferents enter the spinal cord they give off an array of ascending, segmental and descending collateral branches that then enter the spinal grey matter. Some of these collaterals project their activity (through interneurons in various of the spinal grey nuclei) to alpha motoneurons, through which polysynaptic projection system the spinal somatic muscle reflexogenic effects of nociceptive stimulation (involving predominantly facilitation of flexor motoneurons) are generated: whilst others project (again polysynaptically) to the preganglionic neurons of the sympathetic and sacral parasympathetic outflows located in the thoraco-lumbar and sacral segments of the intermediolateral nuclei of the spinal cord, whereby the spinal nociceptive reflex effects on the activity of these outflows are produced.

But more germane to the present discussion is a further group of intra-spinal nociceptive collaterals that penetrate into the dorsal horns of the spinal grey matter, within which many of them run anteriorly to terminate by synapsing on a group of neurons located at the base of the dorsal horn (the basal spinal nucleus, comprising laminae V and VI in Rexed's (1954) classification), the axons of which neurons enter the anterolateral tracts of the spinal cord to ascend into the brain. It will at once be apparent that in order for peripheral nociceptive irritation to evoke the experience of pain in the limbic sectors of the cerebral cortex, the first essential prerequisite is that nociceptive afferent activity entering the spinal cord must depolarize the neurons in the basal spinal nucleus so that they fire up the anterolateral tracts into the brain. Since the extent to which such basal spinal nuclear depolarization occurs will determine (*inter alia*) whether or not pain is experienced (and if it is, its intensity), this basal nuclear synaptic system may be regarded as the nociceptive 'gateway' into the central nervous system; and any neurological mechanism that can modulate the centripetal propagation of nociceptive afferent activity through this synaptic system will have significant effects on the intensity of the resulting painful experience – irrespective of the actual intensity of the evocative stimulation (whether mechanical or chemical) of the tissues nociceptive receptors.

Recent evidence suggests that depolarization of basal nuclear neurons by activation of the nociceptive afferents projecting thereto is effected by release from the synaptic terminals of the nociceptive afferents of a polypeptide transmitter agent (substance P), and that this transmitter release may be indirectly influenced by spinal inputs derived from a variety of peripheral tissue mechanoreceptors (such as those in the skin, muscles and joint capsules) – which mechanoreceptor inputs thereby exert peripheral modulating effects on the experience of pain. As each mechanoreceptor afferent nerve fibre enters the spinal cord through the posterior rami of the dorsal spinal nerve root it gives off segmental and intersegmental collateral branches (amongst many others) that pass into the apex of the dorsal horn and therein terminate on neurons in the apical spinal nucleus (containing lamina II of Rexed (1954)). These apical spinal interneurons then relay the activity reaching them from the peripheral mechanoreceptors into the basal spinal nuclei, wherein the axons of the apical spinal neurons synapse (in axo-axonic synapses) on the presynaptic terminals of the nociceptive afferents – upon whose transmitter release they exert an inhibitory effect. In consequence, then, activity traversing this mechanoreceptor relay system inhibits presynaptically the onward flow of incoming nociceptive afferent activity to the cells of the basal spinal nucleus, and so depresses its centripetal transmission up into the brain at its portal of entry into the neuraxis: and thus it follows that the probability that peripheral nociceptive irritation will evoke the experience of pain (or if it does, the intensity of the experience) will be inversely related to the ongoing frequency of discharge in the mechanoreceptor afferents coming from the affected (or more remote) tissues.

It is for this reason that clinical procedures (some of which are discussed in more detail in later chapters of this book) that enhance the frequency of discharge from tissue mechanoreceptors (such as superficial and deep tissue massage, passive manipulation of joints, or the application to the body surface of tissue vibrators), or which selectively stimulate the large diameter mechanoreceptor afferents in subcutaneous nerves (as do transcutaneous nerve stimulators), will diminish the intensity of many varieties of pain – or even abolish it altogether, if the provoked mechanoreceptor afferent discharge is of high enough frequency and is maintained for long enough. Of course, there is nothing new in the idea that activation of mechanoreceptor inputs may diminish (or even suppress) awareness of pain, since this fact has been an empirically familiar facet of human experience since the dawn of time. Thus every mother knows instinctively that should her child fall over and hurt its knee the appropriate procedure is to massage the injured part and 'rub the pain away'; and again, anyone who bumps his elbow on a hard surface instinctively massages the part to relieve the pain.

But before leaving this matter of peripheral mechanoreceptor suppression of pain, the clinician's attention should be drawn in the present context to the considerable therapeutic effectiveness of the rocking chair in building up massive mechanoreceptor inhibition of nociceptive inputs derived from the lower parts of the body (including the lumbosacral region). Patients with persistent pain in these regions should be persuaded to abandon their customary static chairs for rocking chairs – for as the patient rocks back and forth, the oscillating stresses thereby generated in the skin, muscles and joint capsules in the lower parts of the body produce rhythmic alternating stimulation of the mechanoreceptors located in the stretched and destretched regions of these tissues, resulting in oscillating discharges from their contained mechanoreceptors that gradually suppress the pain through the neurological mechanism outlined above. In fact, there is no better advice that can be given to a patient with lumbosacral or lower limb joint pain (for example) than to 'rock around the clock'.

While much still remains to be done in developing the applications of the experimental data that are already available in the field of peripheral pain research to the specific problems that are presented by the many different varieties of pain that are encountered in clinical practice, there can be no doubt that recognition of the modulating influence of peripheral tissue mechanoreceptor activity upon the centripetal trans-synaptic propagation of nociceptive afferent activity has already proved helpful in a number of circumstances – such as those mentioned above. Furthermore, it may be noted in passing that it now seems that the extreme cutaneous hyperalgesia that afflicts patients with post-herpetic neuralgia is the result of selective viral destruction of the parent dorsal root ganglion cells of the large-diameter mechanoreceptor afferents in the affected peripheral nerves, with consequent loss of their normal presynaptic inhibitory effects on centripetal synaptic nociceptive afferent transmission until (and if) these mechanoreceptor afferent neurons regenerate. A comparable mechanism may underlie the production of the zones of hyperaesthesia that have been observed in the skin of the lower back of some patients with lumbosacral pain, for it may be that in such patients the mechanoreceptors located in the apophyseal joints of the lumbar spine are destroyed (as the result of trauma, or of degenerative or inflammatory diseases involving this region of the vertebral column) and as a result their normal inhibitory effects on nociceptive afferent transmission are lost – although no direct neuropathological evidence of this proposal is yet available. Furthermore, as increasing age in adult life is associated with progressive, selective degeneration of peripheral tissue mechanoreceptors and their large diameter afferent fibres in peripheral nerves throughout the body, the resulting gradual loss of their normal central inhibitory effects on centripetal nociceptive afferent transmission may contribute to the diminishing pain tolerance that characterizes middle-aged and elderly patients, and thus to the greater incidence and severity of non-traumatic pain of various types that is observed in older than in younger subjects. In the present context, it is also relevant to remind clinicians that chronic degenerative neurological diseases (for example, tabes dorsalis) that involve selective degeneration of the dorsal root ganglion cells of the peripheral spinal mechanoreceptor afferent nerve fibres are associated with cutaneous hyperalgesia and episodes of 'spontaneous' pain in various regions of the lower part of the body; and that direct electrical stimulation of the dorsal spinal columns with implanted electrodes – and thus antidromic activation of the ascending collaterals therein derived from peripheral mechanoreceptor afferents – has been found to produce relief in patients suffering from persistent pain, by retrograde (i.e. antidromic) activation thereby of the inhibitory interneurons in the apical spinal nucleus that have already been described.

CENTRAL NOCICEPTIVE PROJECTION SYSTEMS

Ascending spinal nociceptive projections

Should nociceptive afferent activity of peripheral somatic or visceral origin succeed in effecting trans-synaptic excitation of the relay neurons located in the basal spinal nuclei, the efferent discharges provoked therefrom are propagated rostrally into the brain stem in the *anterolateral spinal tracts* – into which the axons of the basal spinal relay neurons pass. In the case of nociceptive projection systems from somatic tissues located caudal to the level of the brim of the pelvis, the basal spinal nuclear axons all cross the spinal cord within the grey matter (obliquely in the anterior grey commissure) to turn upwards into the anterolateral tract on the opposite side of the spinal cord; but in the case of the more rostrally located somatic tissues an increasing proportion of such axons enters the ipsilateral anterolateral tract, so that the spinal nociceptive projection system from such tissues becomes increasingly bilateral from below upwards, (all visceral nociceptive projections – including those from the pelvic viscera – are also bilateral). Furthermore, it should be emphasized that in the human spinal cord the ascending fibres that comprise the anterolateral tracts are spread out over almost the whole of the anterior and lateral segments of the spinal cord, extending from a level anterior to the exiting motor spinal nerve roots to a posterior level that lies dorsal to the plane of the ligamentum denticulatum; and that within each tract its constituent fibres are disposed in somatotopically organized groups in oblique laminae like the segments of a fan, such that those conveying activity from the lower limbs and lumbosacral and pelvic tissues lie (in the supralumbar regions of the spinal cord) lie dorsal and lateral to those transmitting activity derived from more rostrally located tissues. These neuro-anatomical details may at first sight seem to be merely of arcane academic interest; but they are not, for they are vital to the neurosurgeon involved in the performance of anterolateral spinal tractotomies for the relief of persistent pain in various parts of the body – which is why they are mentioned in the context of this chapter.

Before leaving this matter it should be noted that the ascending spinal tract system designated herein as the anterolateral tract is the one traditionally (but as it turns out, erroneously) known as the 'spinothalamic tract'. The latter designation was based on an earlier assumption that all of its constituent fibres ascend without synaptic interruption to the thalamus – but more recent clinical surgical experience and experimental study indicate that this is not so. On the contrary, not more than 30% of the fibres (namely, those of relatively larger diameter and hence of faster conduction velocity) in this tract system actually terminate in the thalamus; most of the remainder are of finer diameter and slower conduction velocity (50–60% of them being unmyelinated) and do not reach the thalamus but instead terminate on neurons in the brain stem reticular system and other brain stem nuclei, whilst still others re-enter the spinal grey matter to synapse on internuncial neurons located therein after ascending for varying distances within the anterolateral tracts. Thus in terms of their operation as a cerebral nociceptive input system, the anterolateral tracts constitute a double-barrelled system – one barrel firing (through a small proportion of relatively fast-conducting, paucisynaptic pathways) into the thalamic nuclei, and the other (larger) barrel firing (through a multitude of more slowly conducting, multisynaptic pathways) ultimately into and through the brain stem reticular system. The clinical significance of each of these components of the spinal nociceptive input system is further considered below.

Nociceptive relays in the brain stem

The fibres in the anterolateral spinal tract system that do not terminate on internuncial neurons within the spinal grey matter (which is most of them) continue their ascent into the medulla oblongata (wherein they lie ventrolaterally near the surface of the brain stem) and mesencephalon (wherein they lie dorsolaterally) (Figure 2).

As each ascending tract traverses the lower brain stem (just dorsal to the inferior olivary nuclei) most of its smaller diameter fibres leave it to enter (as described above) the adjacent longitudinal column of neurons that is the

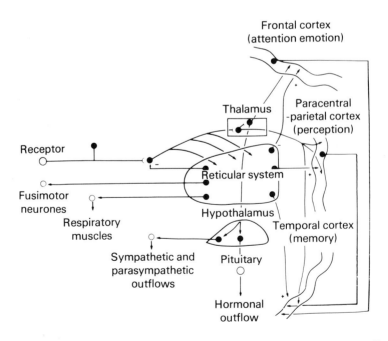

Figure 2 Diagram illustrating the principal pathways pursued by nociceptive afferent activity within the central nervous system. Description and analysis in text

reticular system, while more rostrally others deviate dorsally into the tectum of the midbrain. Much of the activity conveyed in the former (reticulopetal) group of fibres is then propagated further rostrally (and slowly) through a large series of intermediate synaptic relays within the mesencephalic portion of the reticular system ultimately to the centre-median and intralaminar nuclear complexes of the thalamus, whilst activity in the latter (tectopetal) projection is delivered to neurons located in the tectal nuclei.

The remaining small proportion (of larger diameter) fibres ascends still further through the mesencephalon to the diencephalon, finally to enter the thalamus – wherein they terminate on neurons in the posteroventral nucleus, in the intralaminar nuclear system and pulvinar, and in the magnocellular portion of the lateral geniculate body.

The anatomical and physiological observations on the various modes of termination of the fibres in the anterolateral spinal tracts that are summarized above re-inforce the proposal that afferent activity originating in the nociceptive receptor systems located in the peripheral tissues is propagated into the brain to evoke the experience of pain through two parallel pathways – one being a relatively rapidly-conducting, paucisynaptic system that feeds mainly into the posteroventral nucleus of the thalamus, and the other a very slowly-conducting, multisynaptic system whose activity is eventually delivered (via a multitude of intrareticular relays) to the intralaminar and centre-median thalamic nuclear complexes. In this connection, it may be noted in passing that it is much more likely that the familiar dual nature of the experience of pain that follows transient peripheral somatic nociceptive receptor stimulation – the so-called 'fast' and 'slow' varieties of pain – arises from the difference in the time course of transmission of the resulting afferent activity through these two central pathways finally to the cerebral cortex (*q.v.*), rather than that it is due (as the traditional explanation would have it) to differences in the conduction velocity of afferent impulses in two supposedly distinct groups of peripheral afferent nerve fibres that are assumed to be different in diameter from one another – especially since no such clear dichotomy of peripheral nociceptive nerve fibre diameters exists, there being instead (as pointed out earlier) a continuous spectrum of such fibre diameters from 5 μm down to less than 1 μm. Additionally in this context, it should be pointed out that direct electrical stimulation of the anterolateral spinal tract system with appropriately selected stimulus parameters in patients undergoing spinal surgery with local anaesthesia can separately evoke either of these two varieties of painful experience, as a result of selective activation of differing fibre diameter populations within the tract (the few large diameter fibres therein having a lower threshold to electrical excitation than the many more small diameter fibres).

It should also be emphasized that in none of the thalamic nuclear relay sites mentioned above (with the possible exception of the intralaminar nuclei) are there neurons that respond uniquely to peripheral noxious stimulation. Instead, all of them are individually capable of activation as a result either of noxious or of innocuous (*i.e.* mechanoreceptor) peripheral stimulation; and this intrathalamic synaptic convergence of nociceptive receptor and mechanoreceptor inputs on the cells of the posteroventral thalamic nucleus especially may exert a significant influence on the perceptual capacity to localize the peripheral source of pain, as well as contributing to the modulation of its subjectively apparent intensity. Furthermore, neurosurgical experience has shown that in spite of the relatively wide diversity of thalamic nuclei upon which ascending nociceptive inputs terminate (both directly and indirectly), localized surgical lesions placed stereotactically in certain of them (especially the intralaminar and centremedian nuclei) may sometimes result in relief of pain for varying periods of time: and on the other hand, direct electrical stimulation of the same nuclei in unanaesthetized human subjects and animals produces (in the former) pain felt in specific regions of the body and (in the latter) behavioural responses indicative of the experience of pain.

While much still remains to be determined regarding the relative rôles of the different thalamic synaptic relays in generating and modulating the experience of pain, the experimental and clinical data currently available leave little doubt that evocation of this experience depends upon the development of a critical degree of activity in several of the thalamic nuclear systems in response to discharges delivered to them (both directly and indirectly) by way of the central ascending nociceptive afferent pathways projecting thereto – which (in the case of spinally innervated tissues) means the relevant fibres of the anterolateral spinal tracts. But as previously indicated (and as will be discussed in more detail later), generation of this critical degree of activity in the thalamic nuclei depends not only upon the intensity and duration of peripheral nociceptive receptor stimulation but also upon the extent to which centripetal trans-synaptic flow of the afferent discharges resulting therefrom is modulated (in the spinal grey matter and in the thalamic nuclei themselves) by coincident inputs from peripheral tissue mechanoreceptors (as already described) and by the on-going activity of central projection systems to these same synaptic sites (*q.v.*). Nevertheless, once such a degree of activity has been generated in the neurons of the thalamic nuclei it is inevitably dispersed intracerebrally therefrom in four direction simultaneously; and each component of this quadruple extrathalamic projection system makes a specific contribution to the patient's global experience of pain, as follows.

Thalamic nociceptive dispersal systems

Perceptual component
Nociceptive impulses reaching the posteroventral nucleus of the thalamus are relayed thence to (*inter alia*) neurons located in the paracentral (both pre- and postcentral) and inferior parietal regions of the cerebral cortex through fibres that ascend thereto by way of the posterior limb of the internal capsule. The former (paracentral) sector of the cerebral cortex is designated as somatic sensory area I and the latter (inferior parietal) sector as somatic sensory area II, since the ascending inputs thereto are derived from receptor systems located in the somatic tissues – those of contra-lateral origin being directed to sensory area I and those of ipsilateral origin to sensory II so that the cortex of each cerebral hemisphere receives inputs from both sides of the body: activity derived from visceral receptor systems is directed to neurons in the cortex of the insula (island of Reil) on both sides of the brain.

Within the two somatic cortical projection sectors, activity originating in receptor systems embedded in the tissues of the various regions of the body is delivered to radially orientated columns of neurons that are somato-topically organized in terms of the parts of the body from which their inputs are derived – those in somatic area I being disposed cephalocaudally along the central fissure in a latero-medial direction, and those in somatic area II in an antero-posterior direction. Furthermore, within somatic area I afferent activity derived from superficial tissue receptor systems (i.e. those in the skin and subcutaneous tissues) is delivered to cortical neurons that lie closer to the central fissure than those that receive inputs from more deeply located somatic tissues (such as the muscles, joint tissues and periosteum) for instance.

Activation of this somototopically organized thalamocortical projection system underlies the patient's capacity to recognize (with varying degrees of precision) the peripheral anatomical location of the source of his pain and its qualitative nature (i.e. whether pressing, pricking, bursting, stabbing, throbbing or burning), but it does not provoke the experience of pain as such – in other words, nothing hurts in these cortical regions. Thus, experimental peripheral nociceptive stimulation (for example, with thermal stimuli) in the absence of co-incident mechanoreceptor stimulation (a situation, however, that is rare in clinical practice except in respect of pain that is the result exclusively of the chemical abnormalities in tissues that have been described earlier) results in little or no activation of cortical neurons in sensory area I and II, whilst direct electrical stimulation of various parts of cortical sensory areas I or II in unanaesthetized patients never evokes pain – although it gives rise to a galaxy of non-painful somatic sensory experiences in the somatopically related regions of the body. Furthermore, localized traumatic, infarctive or neoplastic lesions involving cortical sensory areas I or II do not impair a patient's awareness of the painful nature of peripheral nociceptive stimulation, although they seriously interfere with his ability to identify its anatomical location – and the same applies with surgical or pathological lesions confined to the posteroventral nucleus of the thalamus from which the paracentral and inferior parietal cortical projection systems arise.

Taken together, then, the above observations indicate that the thalamic projections to the paracentral and inferior parietal regions of the cerebral cortex contribute what may be called the *perceptual component* of painful experiences – that is to say, the sufferer's awareness of whereabouts in his body the source of his pain is located* and his capacity to apply qualitative discriminations to its nature – but nothing 'hurts' as a result of activation of this thalamocortical projection system. Furthermore, this perceptual information appears to be related not so much to the activity derived from irritated peripheral nociceptive receptor systems as to the degree of activity being coincidentally evoked from related tissue mechanoreceptors by the pain-provoking stimulus, which latter activity is transmitted principally through the posterior spinal column–leminiscal system to the same posteroventral thalamic nuclear neurons and thence to the same cortical neurons as receive the nociceptive input from the identical part of the body. This proposal receives support from the clinically familiar fact that the precision of the description of their experience given by patients with pain that involves some element of mechanical irritation is much greater than when their pain is of purely chemical (or visceral) origin; by the fact that the majority of adjectives used by patients in qualifying the nature of their pain are descriptive of mechanical (e.g. 'pressing', 'pricking', 'bursting', 'stabbing', 'throbbing') rather than of chemical (e.g. 'burning') experience; and by the long familiar clinical observation that lesions of the dorsal spinal columns seriously impair a patient's capacity to identify the location and nature of a painful stimulus in the lower part of his body – even though the intensity of his now diffused pain is then often considerably enhanced (*vid. inf.*).

---

*This perceptual localization may sometimes be erroneous (for reasons that cannot be gone into here), as occurs with referred and with phantom pain.

16

Affective component

As indicated at the beginning of this account, the experience of pain is primarily an affective disorder; and evocation of this emotional disturbance is contingent upon activation of a second set of thalamocortical projections; namely, those that pass from the medial, intralaminar and anterior thalamic nuclei to neurons in two regions of the cortex of the frontal lobes by way of the anterior limb of the internal capsule. Within this massive thalamocortical radiation system, it is the fibres in its inferior portion (passing from the dorsomedial nuclei of the thalamus to the orbital surfaces of the frontal lobes) and in its medial portion (projecting by way of the anterior thalamic nuclei to the cingulate cortex) that are of special significance in relation to the evocation of the experience of pain – for it is in the synaptic systems of these two regions of the cerebral cortex that things hurt when nociceptive afferent activity arrives therein.

Within the thalamus, secondary intrathalamic connections link the relay nuclei within which the spinothalamic components of the anterolateral tract system terminate (principally, the posteroventral nucleus) to the dorsomedial and anterior nuclei, and to the intralaminar nuclei (to which reticular projections also pass), from which axons ascend to synapse (*inter alia*) with neurons in the orbitofrontal and cingulate regions of the cerebral cortex – which cortical regions form part of the so-called 'limbic system' that is concerned with emotional experience in general. Nociceptive afferent impulses reaching the thalamus from the peripheral tissues are thus propagated to the orbitofrontal and cingulate regions of the cerebral cortex coincidentally with their delivery to the paracentral, inferior parietal and insular regions of the cortex; and clinical evidence clearly indicates that it is the arrival of such activity in the former regions of cortex that specifically underlies the evocation of the unpleasant emotional experience that is pain – in the present context, then, it might be said that it is in these regions of the brain that things 'hurt'.

For example, clinical study of the effects of selective neurosurgical interruption of the above-mentioned orbitofrontal thalamic projection system in patients with persistent pain – either at its distal end in the operation of orbitofrontal leucotomy or at its origin in the thalamus by the performance of stereotatic thalamotomy – confirms the above proposals. For in either instance, the procedure (when successful) relieves the distress of which the patient complains and his need for powerful analgesic drugs – in other words it relieves his pain, but it does not remove his perceptual awareness of a bodily abnormality. Thus, after such operations the patient remains aware that something is still wrong with a particular part of his body, but no longer complains that it hurts him – the reason being that the surgical procedure has interrupted the thalamic projection into some of the limbic sectors of the cerebral cortex where the emotional experience of pain is evoked, but has left the perceptual projection system (*vid. sup.*) to the cerebral cortex intact. Finally, further emphasis is lent to the validity of the distinction being made here between the emotional disturbance that *is* pain and the perceptual component *of* this experience by the observation that direct electrical stimulation in unanaesthetized patients of the intralaminar thalamic nuclei (which project to the orbitofrontal and cingulate, but not to the paracentral or inferior parietal regions of the cerebral cortex) results in intense unlocalized pain felt in the entire contralateral half of the body.

Memory component

A third (but much smaller) thalamocortical projection system links some of the medial thalamic nuclei (and pulvinar) on each side of the brain to the cortex of the related temporal lobe, in the synaptic circuits of the ventromedial parts of which (with their associated structures) are located the recent and long-term memory storage systems of the brain; and these regions of the temporal lobe also receive secondary inputs from the cortical sectors mentioned earlier through many cortico-cortical association fibres. Thus it is that nociceptive (and mechanoreceptor) afferent activity reaching the thalamus and the limbic and sensory cortical sectors to which the thalamic relay nuclei project (*vid. sup.*) is transferred into the memory-storage system; and it is by this means that a subject builds up his memory of past painful experiences.

Clinical experience and specific neuropsychological study indicate, however, that the efficacy of the transfer of such nociceptive input information from the short-term to the long-term memory storage system is not simply a function of the intensity of individual episodes of painful experience. Instead, the vividness and duration with which the memory of pain is preserved appears to relate much more to the length of time a painful experience lasts (as with chronic painful disorders), or to the frequency with which it is repeated (as with recurrent episodes of acute pain).

Visceral-hormonal reflex component

A fourth (non-cortical) projection system passes from some of the secondary (and especially the medial) thalamic nuclei to the subjacent hypothalamic nuclei located in the ventral diencephalon, which nuclei also receive inputs from (*inter alia*) neurons in the adjacent portions of the brain stem reticular system and (via the amygdaloid nuclei) in the limbic sectors of the cerebral cortex. As the discharges from certain of the anterior and posterior nuclear subgroups within the hypothalamus continuously control the global efferent activity in the parasympathetic and sympathetic outflows from the neuraxis, and as some of the neurons within these same hypothalamic nuclei are also the source of the hypophysoportal hormones that regulate the secretory activity of the adenohypophysis (as well as being the source of the antidiuretic and oxytocic hormones), it will be apparent that the above-mentioned thalamo-hypothalamic projection system provides the principal means whereby nociceptive afferent activity entering the brain evokes the complex of visceral reflex effects (such as those involving the cardiovascular and gastrointestinal systems) and hormonal changes that are inevitably associated with the experience of pain.

Arising out of the above observations, it should be emphasized here – because of the frequent attempts that have been (and continue to be) made to find measurable parameters of physiological function that might serve as so-called 'objective' indices of the intensity of painful experiences – that the thalamo-hypothalamic mechanisms just described operate entirely reflexly in response to nociceptive inputs, and hence the magnitude of the changes in visceral nervous activity and hormonal status thereby produced in patients in pain do not correlate with the intensity of the emotional experience (simultaneously evoked in the synaptic circuits of the orbito-frontal and cingulate regions of the cerebral cortex) that is pain. In short, the visceral and hormonal changes on the one hand and the experience of pain on the other are epiphenomena that are evoked in parallel by the arrival of nociceptive afferent activity in the thalamus, and (for further reasons that will become apparent later) are not directly related quantitatively. Hence clinical attempts to use measurements of changes in pupillary diameter, in heart rate and arterial blood pressure, in electrical skin resistance or skin temperature, or in plasma catecholamine concentration as indices of the intensity of ongoing painful experiences are entirely fallacious – for they are based on the false assumption of a quantitative equation between the hypothalamic reflex effects of peripheral nociceptive receptor stimulation and the cortical affective response thereto. Since a complaint of pain is in essence a description of a subjective emotional state whose intensity is independent of concurrent reflex changes in the sufferer's body, clinically meaningful attempts to assess its severity (or of changes produced therein by various forms of treatment) should be centered on the use of self-rating pain intensity scales based on now well established psychological principles – and not on measurements of concurrent reflexly engendered changes in the state of somatic or visceral tissues, or of alterations in hormonal status.

CENTRAL MODULATION OF PAIN

The quadripartite dispersal within the brain of activity of nociceptive receptor origin that has just been described indicates that each of the thalamic projection systems contributes its own specific component to the global experience of pain. But nowhere within this fourfold intra-cerebral projection system is there any neurological mechanism that can explain the vagaries of the experience of pain that are so apparent to the sufferer in his everyday life. Thus, personal introspective experience reveals all too clearly that the intensity of a pain with which one happens to be afflicted varies widely with one's prevailing emotional mood, with the extent to which one's attention may be engaged by concentration on one's daily tasks, and in response to suggestion by others. Furthermore, experienced clinicians are well aware of the fact that individual patients vary in the intensity of their experience of persistent pain from day to day and from time to time in the course of the day, and that different patients with apparently comparable pathological lesions giving rise to pain may report widely differing degrees of suffering.

Nevertheless, these familiar everyday aspects of the experience of pain have always been ignored or dismissed by those wedded to the traditional (but erroneous) view of pain as a 'sensory modality' whose intensity is directly determined by the activity inevitably provoked in a direct on-line projection system from peripheral 'pain receptors' to a supposed 'pain centre' located somewhere within the brain. Fortunately, however, in recent years a series of neuroanatomical, neurophysiological and neuropharmacological studies has shed considerable light on these clinically important matters, which are especially significant in relation to consideration of the effectiveness of various forms of pain therapy, by revealing that the experience of pain may be modulated up or down in its intensity by concurrent activity in a number of peripheral and central neurological systems that play upon the central nociceptive afferent system at various synaptic stages in its course within the neuraxis.

The clinical implications of the potent peripheral modulating influences that are exerted upon awareness of pain by various tissue mechanoreceptors (and especially those in the skin, muscles and joint capsules) have already been outlined earlier in this chapter. Attention is therefore now directed here to the supplementary modulating effects of several clinically important central projection systems that influence the sequential centripetal propagation within the neuraxis of afferent activity of peripheral nociceptive origin through its synaptic relays in the spinal grey matter, in the thalamus and in the cerebral cortex itself.

Intraspinal nociceptive modulation

The centripetal flow of incoming nociceptive impulses through the gateway synapses in the basal spinal nuclei up into the brain through the anterolateral spinal tracts is modified (additionally to the effects of peripheral mechanoreceptor inputs) through descending projection systems that transmit activity thereto that is derived from neurons located principally (but not exclusively) in the brain stem reticular system, in the medullary raphe nuclei, in the central (periaqueductal) regions of the mesencephalon and in the cerebral cortex.

Reticulofugal modulating system

The major modulating projection system originating from cells belonging to the brain stem reticular system consists of axons of large neurons located medially in its caudal (pontomedullary) region that descend in the dorsolateral tracts of the spinal cord to reach the dorsal horns of the spinal grey matter. Therein they terminate on the apical interneurons whose axons exert the presynaptic inhibitory effects on peripheral nociceptive afferents that have been described previously, upon which apical neurons they exert facilitatory influences and thus (by way of the presynaptic inhibitory effects exerted by these interneurons) produce depression of the transynaptic flow of nociceptive inputs through the gateway synapses of the basal spinal nuclear system. There is some recent evidence (albeit not yet definitive) that this descending reticular facilitation of apical spinal interneurons is affected by release of transmitter dopamine (and/or noradrenaline) from the synaptic terminals of the reticular neurons that are subtended upon the apical spinal neurons; but what is less uncertain is that the apical spinal neurons in the dorsal horn contain high concentrations of one of the small molecular weight encephalins (which are peptide transmitter agents with a chemical structure similar to that of morphine), and that it is release of this opioid transmitter from the synaptic terminals of the apical interneurons onto the nociceptive afferent terminals that is responsible for their presynaptic inhibitory blockade and thus diminution of the awareness of pain. Arising out of these latter proposals, several promising clinical trials have already been made of the use of intrathecal or epidural injections of morphine or meperidine (Pethidine)* for the relief of

*This analgesic effect of spinal injection of meperidine is curious (and at present inexplicable) in the light of the fore-going discussion, in view of the fact that the chemical structure of this drug in no way resembles that of morphine (or of the encephalin transmitter agents).

post-operative pain, and of persistent pain associated with malignant disease – since it is already known that it is at synaptic sites at which the chemically related encephalins function as natural transmitter agents that morphine (and its analogues) exert their familiar analgesic effects.

As this reticulofugal modulating projection system is discharging continuously at varying frequencies throughout life, it will be clear that its activity normally restricts (to varying degrees) the onward flow through the spinal cord into the brain of impulses of peripheral nociceptive receptor origin, thereby re-inforcing the similar effect of inputs from mechanoreceptors located in the same (and related) tissues in depressing awareness of the effects of nociceptive irritation in the peripheral tissues.

The normal (ultimately inhibitory) effect of the activity of this reticulofugal cascade system upon spinal nociceptive afferent transmission is *augmented* when one's attention is diverted away from a painful site in the body by stimulation elsewhere, or by concentration of attention on some particular task; when hypnosis is induced; when hysterical anaesthesia develops; and when the blood concentration of catecholamines becomes very high (as in states of great emotional tension). These facts (*inter alia*) may explain (for example) why distraction of attention, or counter-irritation elsewhere in the body, diminishes awareness of pain; why hypnotic suggestion may be effective in alleviating pain in various parts of the body in some patients; and why soldiers in battle (with consequent high blood concentrations of catecholamines) may sustain severe injuries without being aware of pain. It is also relevant for the clinician to note that numbers of drugs (if administered in individually appropriate doses) may selectively increase the activity of the reticular neurons that operate this inhibitory system, and thereby reduce a patient's awareness of pain without diminishing his general state of alertness; some examples of such drugs are methylamphetamine, chlorpromazine (Largactil) and diazepam (Valium).

Conversely, a *reduction* in the centrifugal inhibitory effect of the caudal reticulospinal projection system on spinal nociceptive afferent transmission enhances the intensity of ongoing painful experiences, and also increases the probability that a particular peripheral tissue stimulus (whether mechanical or chemical) will evoke an attack of pain. Such a situation may arise with exposure to sudden, intense painful stimuli that canalize attention on particular tissues; with specific concentration of the patient's attention on the painful tissues in the absence of distracting stimuli; and following the administration of small doses of ethyl ether or barbiturates. Clinicians should note particularly that it is for this latter reason that patients suffering from chronic pain, or from repeated attacks of episodic pain, should never be given small doses of barbiturates of any type – including quinalbarbitone (Seconal), pentobarbitone (Nembutal) and phenobarbitone (Luminal) – for soporific or sedative purposes, for then the pain will often be intensified to the point where it becomes excruciating agony. Indeed, one of the worst things that can happen to a patient in pain (including postoperative pain) is for some well-meaning doctor to prescribe a barbiturate for him 'to help him get a good night's sleep' – for the exact reverse will often be the case.

Mesencephalofugal modulating system
The grey matter that surrounds the central (Sylvian) aqueduct in the mesencephalon contains (*inter alia*) a dense population of small neurons whose axons descend into the medulla oblongata, wherein they terminate on the cells of some of the raphe nuclei that are embedded in the medulla close to its midline and just deep to its ventral surface. The axons of those raphe nuclei then descend into the spinal cord in the dorsolateral tracts (along with the fibres of the reticulofugal system that has just been described), from which they pass into the spinal grey matter. But having done so, they do not terminate on apical spinal interneurons (as do the reticular projections) but instead appear (at least, as some current evidence suggests) to synapse with the nociceptive relay neurons in the basal spinal nuclei – upon which neurons they exert a post-synaptic inhibitory effect as a result of their release (probably) of transmitter 5-hydroxytryptamine.

Many experimental studies have by now shown that electrical or chemical stimulation of neurons in the periaqueductal grey matter (or in the raphe nuclei) results in inhibition of the transmission of nociceptive afferent activity through the relay nuclei in the spinal grey matter; and more recently, some claims (admittedly of questionable validity) have been made that stereotactic electrical stimulation of the periaqueductal region in patients may produce relief of pain. What now seems very likely, then, is that the pain-suppressive effect of activation of periaqueductal neurons in the mesencephalon is achieved indirectly by virtue of their activation in turn of the medullary raphe nuclei, whose axons descend into the spinal grey matter to produce therein inhibition of the centripetal trans-synaptic propagation of nociceptive afferent activity into the anterolateral spinal tracts.

Of even further clinical interest has been the demonstration that morphine (and other drugs chemically related thereto) produces its clinically familiar analgesic effect partly by activation of this mesencephalofugal system as a result of its stimulation of neurons in the periaqueductal grey matter. Furthermore, it now seems that the sensitivity of these neurons to stimulation by morphine is an expression of their sensitivity to stimulation by opioid-like transmitter peptides that are presented to them naturally from the synaptic terminals (from various sources) that are subtended upon them. These peptide transmitters include at least one of the small molecular weight encephalins and the larger molecular weight β-endorphin – and since the encephalin transmitter in the spinal grey matter produces (*vid. sup.*) presynaptic inhibition of nociceptive afferent terminals whereas the midbrain encephalin results in postsynaptic facilitation of periaqueductal neurons, it seems likely that the encephalin transmitters in these two sites (i.e. in the spinal cord and in the midbrain) differ in chemical structure*.

Arising out of the above observations regarding the operation of this mesencephalofugal modulating system, many proposals (some of them highly speculative) concerning its possible clinical significance for various methods of pain relief (other than by morphine) are being adduced. For example, it has been suggested that the so-called 'placebo' effect (familiar to all clinical pain researchers) that is apparent in 20–30% of all patients in pain who are given dummy medication (or who are provided with dummy physical methods of therapy) results from the fact that these particular individuals react to such procedures with the presynaptic release of increased amounts of endorphin within the central nervous system; and that the rare clinical syndrome of congenital indifference to pain may result from continuous congenital hyperactivity of the central endorphin-producing projection systems. It has also been proposed that the varying degrees of analgesia that may be produced in some individuals by peripheral stimulation with acupuncture needles may involve reflex provocation of activity in these same endorphin-releasing projection systems: on the other hand, however, a few preliminary clinical studies seem to suggest that the production of analgesia by hypnosis does not involve these projection systems.

Corticofugal modulating systems

Neurons in several regions of the cerebral cortex have been shown to exert modulating influences (both facilitatory and inhibitory) upon intraspinal propagation of nociceptive afferent activity. For convenience of description here, these corticofugal modulating systems may be classified as direct and indirect.

The *direct cortical modulating system* is represented by projections from

---

*In this connection, it may be noted that two structurally distinct encephalins have now been identified in pharmacological studies – methionine-encephalin and leucine-encephalin.

neurons located principally in the paracentral and inferior parietal regions of the cerebral cortex that descend, mainly contralaterally, in the corticospinal tract system to terminate in several of the internuncial synaptic relay systems in the dorsal horns of the spinal cord – transmission through which they may facilitate or inhibit. Some of these corticospinal fibres terminate in facilitatory synapses on the interneurons in the apical spinal nucleus, excitation of which leads secondarily (through the relay mechanism described previously) to presynaptic inhibition of nociceptive afferent transmission. Others appear to end in presynaptic inhibitory axo-axonic synapses on the larger diameter mechanoreceptor afferent collaterals subtended on these same spinal interneurons – and activity of these latter cortical projections would then result eventually in enhancement of centripetal transmission of ongoing nociceptive afferent activity.

Whatever the precise functional details of these intraspinal terminations may be, it is now clear that the regions of cerebral cortex to which the 'perceptual' projections of the nociceptive afferent system are delivered exert both negative and positive feed-back influences on the centripetal transmission of activity within this system at the spinal level. These processes may assist in 'sharpening' the subjective localization of the evoc-ative stimulus within the peripheral tissues.

The *indirect cortical modulating system* appears to involve at least two parallel descending pathways – one operating through the caudal reticulospinal neurons that were described earlier, and the other through the endorphin-sensitive neurons in the periaqueductal grey matter of the mesencephalon. The first of these pathways arises from neurons located in several regions of the cerebral cortex – but principally in its superior frontal and parietal regions – that project to the caudal reticular neurons from which the reticulofugal modulating system arises. Some of these corticoreticular fibres exert a facilitatory influence upon the reticulospinal neurons to which they project, and thus (when increasingly excited) enhance reticular blockade of spinal synaptic transmission of nociceptive activity, whereas others have the reverse effect – and several studies in the past decade suggest that variations in the activity of this system (and especially that part of it derived from the superior frontal and anterior parietal regions) may underlie the changes in awareness of peripheral nociceptive stimulation that are associated with alterations in the direction of attention and with induction of hypnosis to which reference has already been made. The second indirect cortical modulating system involves projections that pass polysynaptically (through intermediate relays within the amygdaloid nuclei and the upper reaches of the brain stem reticular system) from neurons in (mainly) the limbic sectors of the cerebral cortex to reach the endorphin-sensitive neurons in the mesencephalon; hence it will be apparent that fluctuations in the activity of this cortico-mesencephalic projection system (resulting, for example, from changes in mood or from peripheral nociceptive irritation itself) will ultimately impose modifying influences upon the intraspinal transmission of ongoing nociceptive afferent activity by way of the mesencephalofugal system described previously.

Intrathalamic nociceptive modulation

Reference has already been made to the fact that transthalamic propagation of incoming nociceptive afferent activity may be modulated therein through the ascending mechanoreceptor relays that converge on the same neurons in the posteroventral thalamic nucleus as do the spinothalamic components of the anterolateral tract system. But additional intrathalamic modulation of the onward flow of such activity may be imposed through projections to the thalamic relay nuclei from neurons in several regions of the cerebral cortex.

These modulating corticothalamic projections – like those entering the corticospinal tracts that have been described previously – arise from neurons located (*inter alia*) in the paracentral regions of the cerebral cortex and descend through the internal capsule to synapse with the postero-ventral thalamic neurons on which the spinothalamic fibres relay – on which neurons they exert long-lasting postsynaptic inhibitory effects. Supplementary postsynaptic (as well as presynaptic) inhibitory effects on thalamic synaptic transmission (through a variety of thalamic nuclei) of nociceptive afferent activity may also be exerted from more widely dispersed cortical neurons located in the frontal, parietal and temporal regions (including the various parts of the cortical limbic system) either through direct corticothalamic projections, or indirectly through subcortical relays to the thalamus via the caudate nucleus (which latter synaptic relays have recently been shown also to involve opioid endorphin transmitter agents).

It therefore seems that neurons located in each of the cortical regions to which centripetal anterolateral spinal tract activity is eventually dispersed to evoke the emotional, perceptual and memory aspects of painful experiences exert retrograde inhibitory influences on the thalamic sites through which such nociceptive activity is relayed to the cerebral cortex, and thereby can 'damp down' awareness of pain. The precise circumstances in which these corticofugal projections to the primary and secondary thalamic relay nuclei operate to modulate painful experiences is still unknown; although loss of their normal inhibitory influence on account of interruption of their pathways by destructive internal capsular or parathalamic lesions (such as may occur in patients with cerebral vascular disease or virus encephalitis, or following intracerebral stereotactic surgery) may have something to do with the production of the syndrome of so-called 'thalamic pain' (syndrome of Déjerine and Roussy).

Intracortical nociceptive modulation

The excitability of the neurons in each of the cortical sectors within which the thalamocortical projections terminate is continuously modulated by ascending activity that reaches them (mainly through relays in some of the so-called 'non-specific' thalamic nuclei) from neurons located in the rostral (and particularly the mesencephalic) portions of the brain stem reticular system, via the reticulocortical projection system. The influence of this continuously-active ascending projection system on cortical neurons is generally facilitatory, so that the excitability of these neurons at any moment is a function of the prevailing frequency of reticulocortical discharge – and for this reason, this system was originally designated as the 'reticular activating system'.

More recent study has led to several modifications of the original anatomical implications of this latter term – but the functional concept of cortical activation provided from neurons located in the upper reaches of the reticular system of the brain stem has been thoroughly validated, in both experimental and clinical contexts.

It now seems that this cortical activating system is operated from rostral reticular and 'non-specific' thalamic (for example, midline and intra-laminar) neurons, and functions as a driving (or 'alerting') mechanism for the synaptic systems within most of the cortical mantle, to which it contributes an unceasing but fluctuating stream of facilitatory impulses. Thus it is that an individual's prevailing global awareness of his environment (that is, his 'state of consciousness'), and the intensity of all his sensory and emotional experiences (including pain), is continuously modulated by the degree of activity prevailing in this system. As nociceptive afferent activity originating in the peripheral tissues is channelled into the brain stem reticular and intralaminar thalamic neuronal systems from the anterolateral spinal tracts (*vid. sup.*), and thereby influences cortical activation through the pathways outlined above, it will be clear that the state of excitability obtaining in the cells of the reticular system (and the related intralaminar thalamic nuclei) at the time when nociceptive impulses are delivered thereto will, from moment to moment, determine the magnitude of the responses of these cells to such an input and thus (through their ascending corticopetal projections) influence the intensity of a patient's experience of pain. In this connection, it is relevant to note that peripheral nociceptive stimulation has been shown to be a particularly potent means of evoking augmented activity in the reticular system and in the cortical activating system.

Experimental and clinical studies extending over the past 20 years have shown that many afferent, metabolic, hormonal and pharmacological influences – too numerous to describe in detail here – may produce moment-to-moment fluctuations in the excitability of reticular and other cortical-activating neurons, and thus in the intensity of the awareness of pain. For example, cortical activation is *enhanced* (and pain is thereby intensified) in states of persisting anxiety; by a moderate increase in the blood concentration of catecholamines; by moderate degrees of hypercarbia (such as obtain in chronic respiratory disease); by the taking of drugs such as dextro-amphetamine (*Benzedrine*), cannabis indica (marijuana) and lysergic acid diethylamide (LSD-50); and by the intake of small amounts of alcohol or caffeine – for this latter reason, therefore, small amounts of alcohol (in the form of brandy or whisky) or caffeine (in cups of tea or coffee) should never be given to patients in pain, as these socially conventional gestures merely intensify the pain. Conversely, cortical activation is *reduced* (and pain is thereby diminished) by emotional tranquility (induced by suggestion, or by the administration of tranquillizing drugs): by hypocarbia (induced by hyperventilation, for instance); by the intake of large amounts of alcohol (which may, in fact, be used as an anaesthetic agent); and by the administration of drugs such as meperidine (*Pethidine*) and the volatile and non-volatile general anaesthetic agents.

As the ascending cortical activating system projects (*inter alia*) to neurons in the orbito-frontal, cingulate, paracentral (and inferior parietal) and temporal sectors of the cerebral cortex, it follows that should afferent impulses from peripheral nociceptive receptors be delivered into the brain at a time when reticulocortical excitability is augmented for any of the reasons mentioned above, the pain will be felt to be intense, it will be relatively well localized within the tissues, and it is likely to be remembered relatively vividly; whereas should the same afferent input enter the brain at a time when reticulocortical excitability is diminished (again for any of the reasons already mentioned) the pain will be felt to be less severe, it will be poorly localized, and memory of the experience is likely to be imprecise and short-lived. In this way, then, the intensity of the emotional experience that is pain, the precision of its perceptual localization within the tissues of the body, and the vividness with which it is likely to be remembered are all conditioned by the degree of activity prevailing in the rostral activating projections to the orbito-frontal, paracentral and parietal, and temporal sectors of the cerebral cortex – and thus (as well as for the several reasons already mentioned) are not solely determined by the physical or chemical intensity of the peripheral nociceptive stimulus. When these observations are added to the other reasons already mentioned, it is hardly surprising that an individual's *pain tolerance* is a widely varying parameter of his experience, and that it bears little relation to his relatively constant *pain threshold*.

Acknowledgements

Grant support for various aspects of pain research from the British Post-graduate Medical Federation of the University of London, the Camilla Samuel Fund, the National Fund for Research into Crippling Diseases, the Clarke Cerebral Diseases Research Trust and the Back Pain Association is gratefully acknowledged.

Bibliography

Detailed reference to the many sources from which the information reviewed in this Chapter is drawn, and to relevant illustrative material, may be found in the following publications (listed in alphabetical order).

Anderson, D. J. and Matthews, B. (eds.) (1977). *Review of Pain in the Trigeminal Region.* (Amsterdam: Elsevier/North-Holland Press)

Barber, J. and Mayer, D. (1977). Evaluation of the efficacy and neural mechanism of a hypnotic analgesia procedure in experimental and clinical dental pain. *Pain.* **4,** 41–48

Beecher, H. K. (1959). *The Measurement of Subjective Responses.* (New York: Oxford University Press)

Black, P. (1970). *Physiological Correlates of Emotion.* (New York: Academic Press)

Bonica, J. J. (ed.) (1974). *Advances in Neurology.* Vol. IV. (New York: Raven Press)

Bonica, J. J. and Albe-Fessard, D. G. (eds.) (1976). *Advances in Pain Research and Therapy.* Vol. I. (New York: Raven Press)

Bonica, J. J., Liebeskind, J. C. and Albe-Fessard, D. G. (eds.) (1979). *Advances in Pain Research and Therapy.* Vol. III. (New York: Raven Press)

Bowsher, D. (1976). Role of the reticular system in response to noxious stimulation. *Pain.* **2,** 361–378

Brodal, A. (1969). *Neurological Anatomy in Relation to Clinical Medicine.* 2nd Edn. (London: University Press)

Cossinari, V. and Pagni, C. A. (1969). *Central Pain. A Neurosurgical Survey.* (Cambridge, Mass.: Harvard University Press)

Critchley, M. O'Leary, J. L. and Jennett, B. (eds.) (1972). *Scientific Foundations of Neurology.* (London: Heinemann)

Dennis, S. G. and Melzack, R. (1977). Pain-signalling systems in the dorsal and ventral spinal cord. *Pain,* **4,** 97–132

Devine, R. and Merskey, H. (1965). The description of pain in psychiatric and general medical patients. *J. Psychosomatic Res.,* **9,** 311–316

Evans, C. R. and Mulholland, T. B. (eds.) (1969). *Attention in Neurophysiology.* (London: Butterworth)

Glynn, C. J., Lloyd, J. W. and Folkard, S. (1976). The diurnal variation in perception of pain. *Proc. Roy. Soc. Med.,* **69,** 369–372

Hilgard, E. R. and Hilgard, J. R. (1975). *Hypnosis in the Relief of Pain.* (Los Altos, California: Kaufmann)

Janzen, R., Keidel, W. D., Herz, A. and Steichele, C. (eds.) (1972). *Pain: Basic Principles, Pharmacology, Therapy.* (Stuttgart: Thieme)

Kerr, F. W. L. (1975). Neuroanatomical substrates of nociception in the spinal cord. *Pain,* **1,** 325–356

Kosterlitz, H. W. (ed.) (1976). *Opiates and Endogenous Opiate Peptides.* (Amsterdam: North-Holland Press)

Krayenbühl, H., Maspes, P. E. and Sweet, W. (eds.) (1976/7). *Pain – Its Neurosurgical Management.* Parts I and II. (Basle: Karger)

Lipton, S. (ed.) (1977). *Persistent Pain: Methods of Treatment.* (London: Academic Press)

Long, D. and Hagfors, N. (1975). Electrical stimulation in the nervous system: the current status of electrical stimulation of the nervous system for relief of pain. *Pain,* **1,** 109–123

Mayer, D. J. and Price, D. D. (1976). Central nervous mechanisms of analgesia. *Pain,* **2,** 379–404

Melzack, R. (1973). *The Puzzle of Pain.* (New York: Basic Books)

Melzack, R. (1975). The McGill Pain Questionnaire: major properties and scoring methods. *Pain,* **1,** 277–299

Melzack, R. and Torgerson, W. J. (1971). On the language of pain. *Anesthesiology,* **34,** 50–59

Merskey, H. and Spear, F. G. (1967). *Pain: Psychological and Psychiatric Aspects.* (London: Baillière, Tindall and Cassell)

Messing, R. B. and Lytle, L. D. (1977). Serotonin-containing neurons: their possible role in pain and analgesia. *Pain,* **4,** 1–21

Nathan, P. W. (1976). The gate-control theory of pain: a critical review. *Brain,* **99,** 123–158

Ray, C. D. and Maurer, D. D. (1973). Electrical neurological stimulation systems: a review of contemporary methodology. *Surg. Neurol.* **4,** 82–90

Sternbach, R. A. (1974). *Pain Patients: Traits and Treatment.* (New York: Academic Press)

White, J. C. and Sweet, W. H. (1969). *Pain and the Neurosurgeon: A Forty Years' Experience.* (Springfield, Illinois: Thomas)

Wyke, B. D. (1969). *Principles of General Neurology.* (Amsterdam and London: Elsevier)

Wyke, B. D. (1974). Neurological Aspects of the Diagnosis and Treatment of Facial Pain. In Cohen, B. and Kramer, I. (eds.) *Scientific Foundations of Dentistry,* pp. 278–299. (London: Heinemann)

Wyke, B. D. (1979). Neurological mechanisms in the experience of pain. *Acupuncture Electrotherap. Res.,* **4,** 27–35

Wyke, B. D. (1980). Neurology of Low Back Pain. In Jayson, M. I. V. (ed.) *The Lumbar Spine and Back Pain.* 2nd. Edn., pp. 265–339. (London: Pitman)

Yaksh, T. L. and Rudy, T. A. (1978). Narcotic analgetics: CNS sites and mechanisms of action as revealed by intracerebral injection techniques. *Pain,* **4,** 299–359

2

Current views on the role of the psychiatrist in the management of chronic pain

I. Pilowsky

INTRODUCTION

The study and treatment of pain has never been one of the central concerns of the pyschiatric discipline, but the situation has changed somewhat in recent years. Probably the simplest explanation for this increased interest in pain is the fact that psychiatric departments are now an accepted feature of the vast majority of general hospitals, and certainly of all teaching hospitals. As a consequence psychiatrists are called upon to provide advice to colleagues in all departments, with regard to the psychosocial aspects of a wide range of physical illnesses. Included among these consultation requests have always been the occasional ones concerning patients with chronic intractable pain. However, until the advent of pain relief clinics such patients were not seen regularly or studied systematically, except by a few psychiatrists and psychologists who were particularly interested.

Once involved with such patients, the psychiatrist has been able to contribute in a variety of ways. These include the classification of pain syndromes, the development of theoretical models for understanding the interplay of cognitive, emotional, personality, social and biological factors; the provision of psychological, behavioural and pharmacological therapies, and the refinement of clinical diagnostic techniques.

THE ROLE OF THE PSYCHIATRIST IN A PAIN CLINIC

The role of the psychiatrist in relation to a pain relief clinic depends to a considerable extent on the setting within which the clinic is operating and, therefore, the type of patients being seen. For example, some clinics may concentrate on the management of terminal patients, while others may see many patients with musculoskeletal problems involving compensation issues. Indeed, those referring patients to a clinic will often be influenced in their referral decisions by their knowledge of the range of personnel available and their interests.

Because of these considerations, it is obviously not possible for precise guidelines to be laid down for the role of a psychiatrist in a pain relief clinic; but what seems quite clear, is that a pain clinic is severely disadvantaged if it lacks ready access to a psychiatrist who has a thorough understanding of pain problems. However, a psychiatrist can only acquire a thorough appreciation of the issues involved as a result of close contact with the entire range of patients presenting to the clinic. This does not necessarily mean that the psychiatrist will take a major role in the treatment programmes of all patients, but he should be able to provide insights which will help to anticipate problems which may arise[1].

A proportion of patients referred to pain clinics suffer from clearcut psychotic and neurotic conditions which require definitive psychiatric treatment. Many, however, show a mixture of emotional and somatic problems which require a range of treatments. A number of such patients can be satisfactorily managed in the psychiatric wards of general hospitals provided that the treatment available includes physiotherapy, occupational therapy, behavioural rehabilitation, and psychotherapy and family therapy, with each modality used as appropriate. In other words treatment directed at physical aspects of the illness should not cease on admission to a psychiatric ward.

A modification of this approach is to set up a 'behavioural medicine unit'. Morgan *et al.*[2] have described such an arrangement; their unit has ten beds and each patient undergoes about five days of diagnostic assessment which includes a traditional psychiatric assessment, physical examination and laboratory tests, a behaviourally oriented interview and psychophysiological assessment and nursing interviews and observation of behaviour. Psychological tests are administered. The treatments used include behavioural techniques, cognitive techniques (use of mental imagery to deal with anxiety and other symptoms), psychophysiological methods (biofeedback) and social skills acquisition therapy. Many problems are treated in this unit of which pain syndromes constitute a significant proportion.

Some pain relief clinics may, of course, have difficulty in arranging for a psychiatrist to make a major commitment to them over a long period of time. Under these circumstances, it might be best for the psychiatrist to be consulted initially on two groups of patients: those in whom a psychiatric syndrome appears to be present, and a fairly random selection of all other patients referred. The purpose of seeking an opinion on the latter group is to provide an opportunity for the psychiatrist and the clinic to discover what his best role might be. In particular, one should not overlook his general educational function vis à vis the other members of the pain relief clinic and vice versa. Above all, it is important that the psychiatric opinion be sought as soon as the patient is referred to the clinic so that his findings can be a part of the data base when the treatment plan is formulated. It is only through such close interdisciplinary collaboration that our understanding of pain is likely to advance.

THE CLASSIFICATION OF PAIN SYNDROMES

From a psychiatric point of view, pain syndromes can be classified according to the standard systems available for psychiatric disorders, or alternatively, within a framework more appropriate to conditions in which the pain complaint dominates the clinical picture.

One useful approach is to group pain syndromes in which psychogenic factors are the chief determinants of the disorder, into those in which the patient is able to accept the fact that such influences are contributing to his illness, and those in which the patient resists any suggestion that the pain is influenced by non-organic factors. In the latter case, we may regard the pain as being a manifestation of 'abnormal illness behaviour'[3a,3b,3c].

Before considering the various forms of abnormal illness behaviour it should be said that pain may be a feature of any psychiatric syndrome. Indeed, the complaint of pain has been found just as frequently among psychiatric as among medical patients[4]. In many such patients, however, the pain is not a prominent feature and the patient may be well aware that psychological stress intensifies the pain. A common psychiatric setting for pain of this sort is a chronic anxiety neurosis, in which case the pain may be regarded as part of a psychophysiological reaction involving particularly muscle tension. Such patients are constantly tense and on edge, alert for environmental threats to an extent which is clearly abnormal. Despite their half-awareness that their pain is dependent on a disturbing life situation, they may be reluctant to offer this view of their illness in the first instance for fear of being criticized or judged weak. However, once the doctor shows his readiness to accept their total situation as a matter for legitimate concern, the patient will be prepared to focus on the psychosocial problems affecting them, and the complaint of pain will recede into the background. The pains complained of by patients with an anxiety neurosis may involve any part of the body but headaches are particularly common and may be described as a constant band-like tightness encircling the head. In patients who also suffer from migraine, it is important to distinguish between tension headaches and true migraine so that the appropriate treatment for each may be prescribed. Apart from pain, these patients will also describe a subjective state characterized by a sense of impending but indefinable danger. They may feel irritable, restless, and the need to be constantly busy. In addition to pain, they may complain of a variety of other physical symptoms such as tremor, breathlessness and paraesthesiae.

Pain may also be associated with depressive neuroses in which the patient usually shows a lifelong tendency to react with excessive despondency in the face of frustrations, disappointments and losses. The patient will appear depressed, refer to himself in self-deprecatory terms and, at times, harbour thoughts of suicide. Such depressive conditions may become chronic, with pain a prominent feature of the illness. As in the case of anxiety neurosis, however, the patient will usually respond to therapy aimed at the psychological problems although he may require some symptomatic treatment for his pain.

Just as pain may occur with neurotic conditions, it may also be associated with psychotic conditions such as endogenous depression and schizophrenia. Indeed, it has been suggested that in both cases pain may somehow alleviate the intensity of the psychiatric syndrome – possibly by providing an acceptable basis for communicating distress to others and thus maintaining interpersonal contact. When pain is prominent in these conditions, it presents special therapeutic and diagnostic problems which are more conveniently discussed within the framework of abnormal illness behaviour (AIB).

ABNORMAL ILLNESS BEHAVIOUR

Illness behaviour may be defined as referring to the ways in which individuals react to aspects of their own functioning which they evaluate in terms of 'illness' and 'health'. The concept of illness behaviour, originally formulated by Mechanic and Vokart[5] has proved an extremely useful framework for considering a number of chronic pain syndromes in which diagnosis and management often prove difficult. These syndromes are characterized by 'abnormal illness behaviour' which is defined as: the persistence of an inappropriate or maladaptive mode of perceiving, evaluating, and acting in relation to one's own state of health, despite the fact that a doctor has offered a reasonably lucid explanation of the nature of the illness and the appropriate course of management to be followed, based on a thorough examination and assessment of all parameters of functioning (including the use of special investigations where necessary) and taking into account the individual's age, educational and sociocultural background.

It will be readily appreciated that abnormal illness behaviour may manifest as either an inappropriate affirmation or denial of illness despite medical advice to the contrary, and that both forms can present severe clinical problems. However, the commoner problem in relation to chronic pain, is that of an inappropriate affirmation of illness and cling-ing to invalidism. Abnormal illness behaviour may be divided into two major forms:

1. Abnormal illness behaviour with predominantly conscious motivation

The main syndromes in this group are malingering and Munchausen's syndrome. Both these conditions are extremely rare and should be diagnosed with the greatest caution. The clue to the presence of such a condition is not simply the discrepancy between complaints and physical findings, but the tendency of the patient to give a 'perfect story'. It should be borne in mind that it is extremely rare for patients to present a text-book description of a syndrome unless they wish the doctor to arrive at a specific diagnosis. In some cases, this may be associated with a wish for access to narcotics, or simply to gain exemption from some unpleasant duty or situation. In some instances, although the patient is conscious of the fact that he is simulating illness, he is not aware of the true motiva-tion for hospitalization and surgical treatment. Where exploration is possible, it may be found that the patient's childhood was an extremely deprived one, with medical contact representing the only experience of caring adults. Such patients often recall periods of illness and hospitaliza-tion as the ony happy events of their early lives.

2. Abnormal illness behaviour with predominantly unconscious motivation

This type of AIB may be divided into neurotic and psychotic forms.

(a) Neurotic abnormal illness behaviour

Obsessional neurosis
Although uncommon, an obsessional concern about the significance of pains may be the major manifestation of an obsessional neurosis. The patient is aware that his fears are ridiculous but cannot drive them from consciousness and repeatedly seeks reassurance. At times the concern appears closer to a delusion rather than an obsession.

Hypochondriacal reaction – phobic type
In this condition the patient is preoccupied with the fear that his pains indicate the impending development of a serious illness. Characteristically he fears that pains in the head mean he is about to have a stroke or develop a brain tumour, while chest pains provoke fears of heart attacks. These patients can at times be reassured, and usually appreciate the fact that their fears are exaggerated and inappropriate; indeed they may even be able to regard their concerns with a degree of wry humour[6].

Hypochondriacal reaction – somatic type
In this form, the patient is constantly preoccupied with his health. His attention is focussed on his pain and its significance. He regards it with a fascinated absorption and worried concern. He considers the various conditions of which it could be a symptom and finds it virtually impossible to accept reassurance although he may be able to do so for short periods. The key feature of this syndrome is the preoccupation with the idea of disease and the absence of any fear of what may happen. These patients are concerned with what they have at present rather than what might befall them in the future.

Conversion reaction
Patients with conversion illnesses present their pain with the same blandness that others may present a hysterically paralysed arm. They usually deny any preoccupation with disease, but focus on their disability and emphasize the distress it causes them. However, they show no depression or anxiety apart from that attributed to disability, and deny any other life stresses.

(b) Psychotic abnormal illness behaviour

Psychotic depression
Where pain is a feature of a psychotic (or endogenous) depression, it may be the focus for a hypochondriacal delusion or it may be a prominent

complaint which tends to obscure the depressive syndrome. When it forms part of a delusional system, the patient may harbour bizarre beliefs, such as the conviction that his bowels are blocked by cancer, or that his bones are crumbling. The key feature is the patient's unshakeable conviction as to the presence of some specific pathological process, in a setting of depressive affect. Where the pain is more prominent, it may sometimes lead to difficulties in detecting the presence of a depressive illness. However, careful exploration of the clinical picture usually reveals the presence of symptoms such as early morning wakening, loss of appetite, loss of libido, and depression, which is often very obvious to the patient's relatives.

Schizophrenia

In the early stages of a schizophrenic illness complaints of pain may be a feature. In some instances, as with psychotic depression, the pain may form part of a delusional system. For example, the patient may believe that his abdominal pain is due to the fact that an electronic device has been implanted in his stomach and that radio waves are being beamed into his body to produce pain. Interestingly, it has been suggested that pain complaints may serve to counter severe personality disorganization in schizophrenia, presumably by providing the patient with a more socially acceptable basis for communicating distress[7].

In some patients, the pain may present as the only symptom and the hypochondriacal or somatic delusion associated with it may be the only evidence for the diagnosis of a schizophrenic illness.

ILLNESS BEHAVIOUR SYNDROMES AND CHRONIC PAIN

As mentioned earlier, while the classification of chronic pain in terms of conventional psychiatric categories is often possible, there are many patients referred to pain relief clinics whose presentations do not fit comfortably into such a framework.

Using the Illness Behaviour Questionnaire (IBQ), Pilowsky and Spence[8] have delineated a number of syndromes in pain clinic patients. The IBQ used in this study was the earlier 52 item version which generates scores for each patient on seven factorially derived scales[9]. These are named: General Hypochondriasis, Disease Conviction, Psychological versus Somatic Perception of Illness, Affective Inhibition, Affective Disturbance, Denial of Problems, and Irritability. The scores obtained by 100 patients referred to a pain relief clinic were classified by numerical taxonomy into six groupings of patients which are described below.

Group 1 patients showed an apparent capacity for using denial effectively. They scored low on all scales and denied any sadness or anxiety. This pattern is not infrequently encountered in patients with terminal neoplastic conditions who tend to communicate only in terms of pain. In some cases their denial may extend to not taking analgesics prescribed for them unless their pain is quite extreme.

Group 2 patients also tend to use denial concerning life problems but do acknowledge some anxiety and depression, suggesting that their use of denial is not completely effective.

Group 3 patients are characterized mainly by their focus on physical ill health, irritability and interpersonal friction.

Group 4 patients show a score profile suggestive of a conversion reaction with somatic focussing and a denial of any other than physical problems.

Group 5 patients report problems in many areas, and resemble masochistic depressive personalities.

Group 6 show high scores on general hypochondriasis indicating a phobic hypochondriasis and also elevated scores on the affective inhibition scale indicating difficulty in communicating their feelings to others.

In order to delineate the illness behaviour which distinguished pain clinic patients as a whole from general practice patients, Pilowsky *et al.*[10] compared two such groups. They found that pain relief clinic patients showed greater disease conviction, somatic focussing and denial of life problems. When pain clinic patients were compared to other hospital patients with painful conditions[8] they differed significantly only on Scale 2, indicating a greater degree of disease conviction, i.e. the pain clinic patients clung more to the idea that they were physically ill than patients with proven physical pathology. It seems, therefore, that what characterizes patients with chronic pain referred to a pain relief clinic is their inappropriate or abnormal illness behaviour. In particular, it is their tendency to use illness behaviour and the clinging to a sick role, as a way of coping. Of course it is not being suggested that all patients with chronic pain are in this category, but certainly a substantial proportion are; and it is in these patients that a psychiatric contribution is most often called for. In order to understand the nature of this form of behaviour, it is necessary to consider the intrapersonal and societal significance of pain.

THE INTRAPERSONAL SIGNIFICANCE OF PAIN

Pain is a universal experience, but since each individual's developmental history is to some extent unique, the concept of pain will inevitably have acquired special meanings for each person.

In the course of childhood pain is associated with two major types of interaction: the receiving of help and care, and the experience of punishment. It has been pointed out that pain and illness behaviour are virtually inseparable[11]. Indeed, Wall[12] in a masterly consideration of the pain experience has proposed that it is more appropriate to regard pain 'as an awareness of a need-state than as a sensation', and that 'pain signals the existence of a body state where recovery and recuperation should be initiated'.

It will be readily appreciated that the degree to which pain plays a role in gaining care and attention for a young child will greatly influence the extent to which pain (and therefore, illness behaviour) achieves a prominent role in the repertoire of coping strategies. In this way any form of distress, whether it be anxiety or depression may be communicated through pain statements. Indeed, by mobilizing memories of caring responses to such behaviour the unpleasant affects may be alleviated without the need for the response of another person, since the pain experience may allow the individual to withdraw attention from others and lavish care on himself.

In certain families care and affection may only be provided in the context of pain. Thus a child may only really be given attention after it has been punished physically. The impression may thus be conveyed that the child is basically bad and can hope to attain love only following expiation by punishment.

One of the most illuminating descriptions of the intrapsychic significance of pain has been provided by Engel[13]. This author delineated the characteristics of what he described as the 'pain-prone patient' based on his clinical experience over a period of fifteen years. He reports that guilt is almost always a factor in the choice of pain as a symptom. (Indeed, it is interesting to reflect on the fact that it is rarely possible to experience pain and guilt simultaneously – it appears as though a quantum of guilt is always neutralized by a quantum of pain.)

Chronic pain patients are commonly guilt ridden, depressed and possessed of low self-esteem. In female patients a recurring pattern is that of a family history involving a mother who was chronically ill throughout the patient's childhood, often with pain as a prominent symptom. In some cases, the pain may even be attributed to the patient's birth. It is not surprising therefore, that such individuals may be chronically burdened with guilt and tend unconsciously to manoeuvre themselves into situations which are bound to cause them pain and humiliation.

Engel[13] also described a history of family aggression both verbal and physical, between parents and directed at their child. He found that patients often had their first attack of pain during adolescence. Thereafter attacks occurred when their need to suffer was not satisfied by external events. Thus a patient might report that the pain had begun 'just as everything began to go well for the first time'. In addition, pain may occur as a response to a real or threatened loss of a significant person or possession. Indeed, the painful part may symbolize the lost person and at times have the precise characteristics of a pain suffered by that person. At the same time, the pain experience allows the sufferer to expiate the guilt over the sorts of aggressive feelings towards the deceased so often present during grief states.

We see then that within the individual, pain may serve several important functions which contribute to the attainment of psychological equilibrium. In particular, it helps to deal with guilt over feelings and ideas felt to be unacceptable or wrong.

THE INTERPERSONAL SIGNIFICANCE OF PAIN

At the interpersonal level, pain has a number of effects once it is communicated by either verbal or non-verbal means.

In the first place, the communication of a pain state may serve to control the behaviour of others. It directs their attention to the sufferer and away from other matters. In this way it may lead others to gratify the patient's need to be dependent and cared for. But it may also serve to punish others indirectly, by depriving them of the attentions of the person who is now occupied with the needs of the individual in pain.

Pain also allows the individual to withdraw from the company of those whom he wishes to avoid for whatever reason. Since it generally confers the privileges of the sick role it may permit the overt display of irritability and rudeness without the usual retaliation such behaviour might normally provoke.

Finally, pain complaints may allow the covert gratification of sexual drives in those who find such impulses anxiety provoking. Thus pain allows attention to be turned to the patient's body and others are drawn into transactions involving physical contact. In this way patients may derive considerable guilt-free sexual pleasure from their encounters with doctors in much the same way as small children use the enactment of 'doctor and nurse' games to explore each other's bodies. Indeed, in order to obtain the guilt-free pleasure of being close to a doctor of the opposite sex the patient may be prepared to undergo many painful and uncomfortable procedures.

The response to the patient's pain of those close to him may take many forms since pain evokes a wide range of feelings and behaviours in others. Initially, they may respond with concern and a fear of losing the individual in pain. Care is provided and measures taken to provide comfort and help. There may, however, also be feelings of anger and associated guilt, if the pain persists and produces inconvenient and difficult consequences for family members. These feelings of anger and guilt may provoke negative reactions to the sufferer, and a withdrawal from him. In some cases, however, the guilt feelings may result in more help being provided than the patient requires.

Some family members may actually encourage illness behaviour and invalidism in the pain sufferer. Apart from being a manifestation of a reaction formation to an unconscious wish to punish the patient, this type of attitude may stem from the fact that the relative derives vicarious gratification by identifying with the person receiving help and support. In addition, some individuals feel secure only when someone else is dependent upon them. Under such circumstances the relative feels that there is little likelihood of abandonment and that their situation in life is more secure with an invalid in their care. It can readily be appreciated that in this way both the pain sufferer, and the family may become locked into a pathological relationship which satisfies both their neurotic needs.

On occasion the advantages to a family may be of a more tangible nature, in that the pension or compensation received by the patient may be of considerable importance to its survival. However, this is rarely a significant reason for the family's tendency to reinforce the patient's invalidism[14].

THE SOCIETAL RESPONSE

At a time when most societies make substantial contributions to health care systems any symptom which is chronic and demands the allocation of limited resources, constitutes a problem of some magnitude. This is the case particularly when the degree of suffering and disability is difficult to establish 'objectively', i.e. on the basis of demonstrable organic pathology, as often occurs in the case of chronic pain. This issue causes difficulty in compensation cases where there is invariably a concern that the individual seeking redress may be malingering. Increasingly, however, it is being appreciated that malingering is uncommon and that the factors operating in chronic pain and disability following industrial and other accidents, are extremely complex.

PERSONALITY AND CHRONIC PAIN

Thus far the role of pain in relation to dynamic intrapersonal and interpersonal processes has been described. We now turn to studies which have sought to delineate personality patterns associated with chronic pain, using psychometric methods. In particular, attention has been focussed on differences between patients with and those without a clear organic element to their pain.

Woodforde and Merskey[15] studied 43 patients referred for psychiatric consultation of whom 27 were regarded as having an organic cause for their pain, while 16 lacked such evidence. The patients where asked to complete the Middlesex Hospital Questionnaire and the Eysenck Personality Inventory. The results obtained indicated that both the 'organic' and 'psychological' groups achieved scores similar to those of psychoneurotic outpatients. High scores for presence of phobias and obsessionality occurred in the male group of those with organic lesions. In addition, it was found that the organic group had a higher L score on the Eysenck Personality Inventory, indicating a tendency to 'fake good'. The authors suggest that this tendency could be a manifestation of a response to chronic distress and a fear of showing weakness. It is extremely interesting that in this study those classified as organic were found to score in a neurotic direction. It may well be that this was due to the fact that the more anxious and neurotic patients had been selected by those who referred them for psychiatric assessment.

In a study of the personality traits of psychiatric patients with pain, Merskey[16] gave the Maudsley Personality Inventory to three groups: psychiatric patients with pain, psychiatric patients without pain, and normal controls. Surprisingly, he found that the patients with pain had slightly lower neuroticism scores than those without pain. He also found that there was a tendency for patients with pain to have a higher extraversion score than those without pain, and especially than those with depression. This finding is in keeping with the study reported by Bond[17] who found association between higher extraversion scores and a tendency to complain of pain. In this regard, of course, it is important to be aware of the distinction between the experience and the communication of pain. In other words while certain factors may determine the nature of the pain experience, others may play a larger part in deciding the ways in which the pain is communicated to others.

There are obvious advantages associated with the study of personality and pain in certain specific pain syndromes. A number of studies have been carried out to delineate the personality associated with chronic low back pain.

Sternbach and his co-workers[18] reported on a series of over 100 consecutive patients seen at a low back clinic. When compared to patients with rheumatoid arthritis, these patients were found to have significant depression, a life-style of invalidism, and a tendency to engage in 'pain games'. It was not possible to establish what the precise temporal relationship of the depression had to the pain, but on the Minnesota Multiphasic Personality Inventory (MMPI), these patients scored on average two standard deviations above the normal mean on the depression scale. They found an even more prominent degree of hypochondriasis consisting of a somatic concern and preoccupation with symptoms. The 'pain games' to which these authors refer include a tendency to challenge doctors to diagnose and relieve the pain but, at the same time, to resist in a variety of subtle ways all efforts to achieve this end.

Gentry *et al.*[19] studied 56 patients manifesting chronic low back pain of whom 31 where male and 25 female. All these patients had been referred by the orthopaedic department for routine pyschodiagnostic evaluation. They had all had one or more spinal operations in addition to other treatments, and had nonetheless continued to experience pain and disability for long periods of time. The average period since first onset of symptoms was 7.5 years for the entire group, and ranged from a few months to 40 years.

The patients tended to deny any emotional problems, and manifested marked somatic concern. Their major psychological defence mechanisms were denial and repression. Although they gave an appearance of being extroverted and sociable, there was evidence that they were self-centred, demanding and dependent. Other tests demonstrated that these patients placed emphasis on family cohesion and reference to parents and spouses tended to be positive. On the other hand, reference to unpleasant feelings, such as anger, were conspicuously avoided.

The authors' observations regarding the developmental history of such individuals are extremely revealing. Their findings indicate that most patients had unsatisfactory childhoods in the sense that their dependency needs were not properly met. They were the later children in large families and started work early, in relatively hard jobs. They, in turn, married early and had several children of their own. The authors feel that these individuals tend to postpone the gratification of their own dependency needs until an injury, which provided an acceptable means of depending on others for support in both the emotional and economic sphere of their lives.

A further significant finding was that in many of these patients, models for pain and disability had been present during their childhood. In other words, they had been associated with one or more parents who had complained of pain and disability over a long period of time. The authors emphasize that no single factor can be regarded as a major determinant of chronic low back pain. In addition, their findings underline the fact that malingering is very uncommon in this group of patients.

McCreary et al.[20] investigated the differences between low back pain patients who showed organic pathology and those who did not. They compared 42 patients who were classified as organic, and 37 who were classified as functional, on their responses to the MMPI. They found that the functional low back pain patients had higher scores on the hypochondriasis, hysteria, psychopathic deviation, schizophrenia, mania and social introversion scales. However, they emphasize that the degree of overlap was high and that personality data should be used with extreme caution in attempts to separate groups of patients in a low back pain population.

Leavitt et al.[21] carried out a similar study in low back pain patients, but focussed mainly on the descriptions of pain provided by the patient groups. Their chief finding was that the pain described by the patient with an organic lesion was consistent and specific, while the patients without evidence of organic pathology gave descriptions which were more variable and diffuse and they reported more intense pain.

Another approach to the understanding of low back pain is to consider the effect of psychological factors on the response to operative intervention. Blumetti and Modesti[22] studied 24 females and 57 males with chronic low back pain. Of these, 8 females and 34 males were treated with methods such as rhizotomy, cordotomy and transcutaneous stimulation. They found that the patients who were unimproved by treatment scored higher on the hypochondriasis and hysteria scales of the MMPI, and the symbiosis scores on the projective tests. Those who responded to treatment were less preoccupied with bodily concerns and, also, less dependent on others; in addition, they were less rigid in terms of their defences and consequently did not need to rely simply on somatic complaints to cope with the world around them.

Spring et al.[23] studied 35 patients with low back pain due to disc protrusion, pre- and post-operatively. They found that 30% developed new pain syndromes after the operation, and concluded that neurotic problems may persist or intensify post-operatively. They stressed the need to provide therapy for the psychological aspect of patients' problems, in addition to the physical component.

Lloyd et al.[24] carried out a study of 188 patients who had been referred to a rheumatology outpatient clinic for persistent low back pain. (Patients with pathology such as ankylosing spondylitis, neoplasm or direct trauma were excluded from the study.) They were treated along conventional lines, and categorized on the basis of their response to treatment. Patients who were still attending after 90 days were regarded as suffering from persistent low back pain and were given more intensive psychiatric investigation. Of the original patients seen, 135 completed Middlesex Hospital Questionnaire forms and these were used to find predictors of outcome by comparing the profiles of patients who had been discharged with those who had defaulted or were regarded as persistent. It was found that patients who defaulted had higher hysteria scores than those in the other two groups, and patients who were discharged tended to be older. Of the patients with persistent back pain, 8 had depressive neurosis. On the basis of their findings, the authors conclude that patients with persistent low back pain who may require psychiatric treatment can be detected when first seen if evidence of a depressive disorder is searched for. It would have been extremely interesting, however, to know more about the patients who defaulted in view of their higher hysteria score at the beginning. It is quite possible that their low back pain also persisted, but that for some reason, they did not find the rheumatology clinic suitable for their needs.

Studies of patients with chronic pain affecting the head and neck, have revealed personality characteristics which, in some cases, overlap those of patients with low back pain. Gross and Vacchiano[25] studied 59 females with temporomandibular joint dysfunction whom they compared with controls, using Form A of the 16 Personality Factor Questionnaire. They found that patients with temporomandibular joint dysfunction tended to be conventional and concerned with immediate issues. They lacked frustration tolerance and tended to worry. They were generally dissatisfied, phobic, hysterical and obsessional. They also reported sleep disturbances, and showed low ego strength and higher superego (conscience) activity.

Daniel Lupton[26] reported on a study of 200 patients complaining of craniofacial pain. When these patients were compared with a variety of control groups, including other dental patients, medical patients suffering from arthritis, healthy women, and psychiatric patients, they showed some interesting personality characteristics. Thus they tended to describe themselves, (and were described by others) as responsible, generous and managerial. They appeared to depend heavily on denial and repression to maintain a self-concept which reflected normality and independence. Under these circumstances it seemed that they were able to complain only of physical problems in order to reveal distress. Lupton[26] reports that the psychological factors associated with non-organic temporomandibular joint dysfunction, respond to treatment and that this results in relief of physical symptoms as well. He points out that best results were obtained with patients who had been managed conservatively by the first doctor they saw, and who were given clear information about the psychology and physiology of their complaint. Those who did worst had been promised complete cures, and when this did not eventuate they became increasingly disillusioned and resentful.

An interesting psychiatric aspect of a typical facial pain has been described by Delaney[27] who reported on three women who were seen with psychotic symptoms shortly before projected neurosurgical therapeutic procedures. They were hospitalized and treated with major tranquillizers, which resulted in relief of both the pain and of the psychotic symptoms. Two of the patients were followed up for twelve months and showed no return of either psychiatric or pain symptoms. Delaney[27] suggests that in these patients the chronic pain was serving as a defence against the psychotic illness.

A relatively uncommon symptom in pain relief clinics, but one not unfamiliar to dentists is that of chronic orolingual pain, or 'burning mouth'. Schoenberg and his coworkers[28] reported on a series of 21 patients with this syndrome. Of these 81% were regarded as clinically depressed, while the others also showed evidence of covert depression. The authors noted that the symptom was often related to a significant loss. On the MMPI they showed high scores on the depression scale. Two of the patients were overtly schizophrenic and in others there was evidence of diffuse hypochondriacal concerns apart from the burning mouth. On the basis of their findings, the authors concluded that the treatment of depression was extremely important in the management of this condition.

PATHOPHYSIOLOGY OF CHRONIC PAIN

An interesting aspect of chronic musculoskeletal pain concerns the role of physiological changes in contributing to the pain. In this regard, Moldofsky and his co-workers[29] have carried out a series of interesting studies into the 'fibrositis syndrome'. They have shown that patients with this condition complain of disturbed sleep and stiffness and pain on waking. When their EEG patterns were studied through the night, they showed the presence of alpha rhythms in non-REM sleep. The same complaints were produced in six normal males by depriving them of stage 4 sleep. On awakening they complained of stiff, sore muscles, lower pain threshold and mood disturbances. On the other hand, three very fit males who were deprived of stage 4 sleep did not develop symptoms. The authors suggest that there may be an internal arousal mechanism operating in competition with the non-REM sleep system. They speculate that this may stem from psychological distress, and the fibrositic symptoms may be secondary. They also postulate that a defective serotonin metabolism might produce both the sleep disorder and the fibrositic symptoms. In a further study, Moldofsky and Walsh[30] investigated plasma tryptophan in eight patients with the fibrositis syndrome. They found that the plasma-free tryptrophan level was inversely related to the severity of subjective pain. This finding is consistent with the theory that there is a relationship between decreased brain serotonin metabolism and pain reactivity.

Similarly, muscle tension has been shown to be associated with patients complaining of muscle contraction headaches. Vaughn *et al.*[31] studied ten subjects with frequent tension headaches and ten controls. They exposed all subjects to the stress of mental arithmetic and found that the frontalis electromyograph of the headache group showed higher pre-stress activity. There was also a greater change in frontalis activity after stress in the low-frequency headache group. There was a significant correlation between the perceived level of relaxation and the electromyograph in the low frequency group but not the high frequency headache group.

In a related study van Boxtel and Roozeveld[32] were able to show that frontalis EMG activity was associated with muscle contraction headaches. They studied the EMG frontalis, temporalis, trapezius and

47

forearm muscles during a mental arithmetic test in seven subjects with muscle contraction headaches and eleven controls. They found that the frontalis activity differentiated between the two groups. Both these studies indicate the importance of muscle activity in the experience of chronic pain.

PSYCHIATRIC ASPECTS OF CHRONIC PAIN

These findings raise interesting issues with regard to the treatment of pain. Studies referred to this far indicate the presence of personality difficulties, depression and an attempt to cope with problems by the use of physical symptomatology. It is relevant to consider a number of recent studies which have been carried out in psychiatric patients, to elucidate some of the associations between pain and psychiatric illness.

Delaplane *et al.*[33] studied 227 patients admitted to a psychiatric hospital; pain was complained of by 86 of these but in only 27 could a physical cause be demonstrated. A comparison with other patients indicated that women were more often affected by pain and tended to complain of more severe pain. Men were more likely to have a physical diagnosis, usually involving low back pathology. The presence of pain was associated with the diagnosis of anxiety states and personality disorders. The authors concluded that pain is a relatively common symptom in psychiatric patients and its aetiology is emotional in many instances.

Merskey and Boyd[34] investigated 141 patients with chronic pain of whom 71 showed evidence of an organic cause and 70 did not. They found less evidence of childhood family disturbance in those with organic pathology, and fewer premorbid personality problems and neurotic traits. Pain described as psychogenic was associated with the experience of punishing mothers and rejecting fathers.

A study which helps to clarify the relationship of pain and depression was carried out by Mohamed, *et al.*[35]. They studied 13 patients with depression and persistent pain, and a control group of 13 matched subjects with depression and no pain. They found that the patients with depression and pain reported more severe depression. They also had a greater number of pain problems in the past, more pain problems in their spouses and families, as well as pain problems in the families of their spouses. There was a consistency in the location of pain between patients and their spouses and between patients and their spouse's family. The pain group showed more marital maladjustment. The authors conclude that the location of pain might be influenced by the experience of pain in some significant person in the patient's life.

Although it can be seen that certain consistent themes relating to personality functioning and psychiatric symptomatology have emerged in a number of studies, these findings must be interpreted with caution since they may be influenced by selection factors. In this regard, the study of Pilowsky, *et al.*[10] referred to earlier, is of some interest when compared with that of Chapman, *et al.*[36] Thus, in the former study 100 patients referred to a pain relief clinic were compared with 78 patients attending the family medicine unit practice of the same hospital. All patients completed the Illness Behaviour Questionnaire and the Levine–Pilowsky Depression Questionnaire (LPD). Pain clinic patients achieved higher scores on depression, general hypochondriasis, disease conviction and affective disturbance. They also showed significantly greater tendency to somatize their complaints. In the subsequent study, Chapman *et al.*[36] compared 200 pain relief clinic patients with 200 patients referred for the treatment of pain to a private practice clinic. They found that the private practice patients scored lower on general hypochondriasis, disease conviction and affective disturbance, and also showed less tendency to somatize. These patients also achieved a lower score on the LPD depression scale. These findings indicate that the characteristics which emerge in chronic pain patients referred to a pain clinic cannot be generalized to all patients with persistent pain.

THE MULTIDISCIPLINARY APPROACH TO TREATMENT

The findings with regard to the personality and emotional status in patients with chronic pain makes abundantly clear that any treatment approach must take into account the patient's personality and social situation, and direct some aspects of the treatment to these areas. This approach has been adopted by the large number of multidisciplinary pain clinics which, in recent years, have undertaken the management of intractable pain. Since a considerable range of expertise is required in such pain relief clinics, most include anaesthetists, neurosurgeons, neurologists, occupational therapists, physiotherapists, psychiatrists, and psychologists. The emphasis in such clinics is on the multimodal approach to the pain problem. A central issue in the management of chronic pain is that although psychological factors may be contributing in large measure to the pain experience, it must be realised that, as many studies have shown, the patient's illness behaviour constitutes virtually his only defence against his inner conflicts. Thus, any treatment which implies a rejection of the patient's status as someone with a physical illness is extremely threatening and may cause a worsening of the illness or withdrawal from the treatment programme. For this reason in the majority of the patients, psychotherapy is only likely to be effective if associated with treatments directed at physical discomfort. It is probably only in this way that patients can feel assured that others regard their pain as 'real'. It should be borne in mind that patients who say that others do not regard their pain as 'real' are often projecting their own attitude onto those around them. This is not to say that many of those they encounter in hospitals may not regard their pain as imaginary, but that they, themselves, can probably recall having adopted the same attitude towards other pain sufferers in the past. When questioned about this, pain patients will usually admit to this fact and, indeed, confirm that they themselves have often wondered whether they were imagining their own pain. Thus, the need to establish that the patient's pain is real is extremely important but, at the same time, it is necessary to see that this concern over the reality of the pain is more complex than it might appear at first sight. A further and extremely important point, is to distinguish between pain, illness behaviour and disability. Patients may report pain and show abnormal illness behaviour while, at the same time, not be as disabled as one might expect them to be. In fact, it is not unusual to find patients who complain of severe pain also reporting an extremely busy life, often undertaking tasks which are calculated to make pain worse.

A number of centres have begun to report on their methods of managing chronic pain and the results they have achieved. Cairns and his co-workers[37] have described a treatment programme for the management of chronic low back pain. Patients are initially seen in the outpatient department where a full history and examination are carried out and the Cornell Medical Index is administered, as well as a daily activity schedule. On the treatment unit there are two distinct phases. First, there is an orthopaedic evaluation which includes regional blocks if required and narcotic and psychotropic medication as necessary. In phase two, the patient is treated in the operant conditioning unit as an inpatient for 4–6 weeks. The operant conditioning approach[38] involves encouraging the patient to complain less of pain and to involve himself in increasing amounts of activity by responding less and less to manifestation of illness behaviour and encouraging and reinforcing increased amounts of activity. The patient's activity programme is changed each day, and the amount of time spent out of bed is displayed on a graph on the wall of his room. The amount of praise and attention and desirable conversation depends on the amount of improvement the patient shows. A particularly interesting aspect of the programme is the fact that the amount of time the patient spends out of bed is recorded electronically by a device which displays visually whatever he achieves.

In addition to the behavioural approach the patient is asked to set goals for his life after discharge. These include vocational, domestic and recreational objectives. Throughout the patient's stay, he is involved in group discussions which family members attend. After discharge, patients were followed-up by mail; the average follow-up was 10 months and of the 100 patients surveyed 90 responded. The results indicated that 70% improved and 74% had not sought further treatments. Of those given vocational training, 75% were working at follow-up or were involved in a training programme. Despite the short-comings associated with postal follow-up methods, these results are clearly encouraging.

Ignelzi *et al.*[39] reported on the results of a follow-up of 54 patients who had been treated in a multidisciplinary programme. This programme included vocational rehabilitation, physical therapy, operant conditioning, relaxation therapy, and group therapy. The follow-up period was between 2 and 3 years. Patients reported significantly less pain, reduced analgesic intake, and increased activity levels. No differences were found between those who had been treated surgically and those who were not operated on. Newman *et al.*[40, 41] have also reported encouraging results in the treatment of low back pain patients in a multidisciplinary centre. They conceptualize pain in terms of seven overlapping models: the sensory, psychodynamic, operant, economic, interpersonal, cognitive and psychophysiological elaboration models. The sensory model highlights the pathophysiological component of pain. The psychodynamic model leads to an understanding of the way in which unconscious impulses may produce pain as in conversion hysteria and, also, raise the question of secondary gain. The operant model focuses on the pain behaviour which can be controlled by contingent rewards or punishment. Economic models point out that pain may constitute a solution to a personal problem and in this sense, relate to the psychodynamic approach. The interpersonal model leads to a description of the communication value of pain and its effect on others. The cognitive model draws attention to the patient's beliefs and expectations about his health, and the meaning of the pain he experiences. The psychophysiological elaboration model proposes that chronic pain leads to physiological changes which result in a worsening of the pain experience and disability.

Using this theoretical framework, Newman et al.[41] treat patients over a 3 week period, after a complete evaluation and educational session. New patients are encouraged to relate to patients who have been in the centre for two or three weeks, using them as role models. The programme encourages self-help by providing physical therapy, a graduated exercise programme, biofeedback, relaxation training, psychotherapy, communications training, conjoint and family therapy. As far as possible, the patient is encouraged to become responsible for the control of his pain. Most are taught how to use a transcutaneous nerve stimulator and it is found at follow-up that these tend to be used less and less. Every attempt is made to understand the patient's psychodynamics as well as the family's interaction pattern, but intensive psychotherapy is not undertaken. In fact, such an approach is not particularly acceptable to their chronic pain patients. The operant approach influences most staff attitudes to the patient so that when desirable behaviour is manifested they provide increased amounts of attention. Analgesic medications are not given on request, but rather on a scheduled basis. 'Psychophysiological imbalances' are treated with biofeedback therapy and relaxation. In an 80 week follow-up of 36 patients with low back pain, it was found that there was a reduction of analgesic use and an increase in physical functioning. Interestingly, although reports of pain persisted, medical resources were used less.

The results of a very similar programme have been reported by Swanson, et al.[42] Their 200 patients were rather typical of those referred to pain relief clinics with many years of pain, multiple operations, treatment failures, disability, compensation factors and dependency on medication. At the time of discharge, 59% were moderately improved or better. At 3 months, 40% were still doing well, and at one year 25% were doing well. Thus, at one year 65% of the original successes were still well. The purpose of this programme is to help the patient and family cope, to reduce medication and, if possible, to reduce pain. Behaviour modification is central to the programme which also includes physical rehabilitation, education, family participation and psychological therapy. Videotape feedback is used in order to demonstrate the patient's behaviour to himself. He is also required to record on a graph his subjective pain, his active time and any other specific physical achievements. Medication is given on request at first, but thereafter at fixed times in a masking vehicle and with gradual reduction of the dose. Psychotherapy is of the supportive type. It is important to appreciate that only patients who accept the programme are accepted and it is designed for those for whom no medical or surgical alternative is available. The authors state that the programme is not suitable for patients with unrealistic expectations, psychoses, severe drug dependency or extensive medico-legal complications.

Swanson et al.[43] have also described the characteristics of patients who registered formal complaints about the management programme. They studied records of 30 such individuals and found them to be among the most chronic and unresponsive to therapy. They had problems of dependency on medication, accident proneness, and reported dissatisfaction with previous treatments. They opposed any psychological approaches to their illness, and in some cases, manifested circumscribed delusions. Of the 13 patients, 12 were female and more than half were unmarried. They had longer periods of pain, more time off work, more hospitalization and operations. Six of the patients were deluded about the causes of their pain, medical findings and staff attitudes, as well as society's response to their pain. They gave a history of a traumatic childhood and adolescence, with a psychiatric history. They had marked conflicts over dependency, and more than 4 years impairment of capacity for work. The study suggests that these patients are, in a sense, caricatures of chronic pain patients, and it is clearly important to recognize them very early. These patients generate marked staff reactions characterized by feelings of anxiety, guilt and anger. The authors suggest that when this syndrome is diagnosed early, patients can be allowed to observe the programme before commiting themselves to it.

Maruta, Swanson and Finlayson[44] examined 144 patients with chronic pain of non-malignant origin and found that 24% were drug dependent, 41% drug abusers, and 35% were non-abusers. The drugs most commonly used were codeine and oxycodone. The authors differentiated between abuse and dependency on the basis of World Health Organization and other criteria. The essential difference seemed to be that drug dependency implied a greater degree of narcotic use. The interesting aspect of this study was that on most of the measures used, very few differences emerged between the three groups of patients. The authors believe that this may be due to the fact that there is so much psychopathology present in the pain clinic group as a whole, that differences related to the use of drugs are not easy to detect. They emphasize, of course, the need to detect drug dependency as early as possible in treatment so that it may be properly managed.

In contrast to the above studies, Katami and Rush[45] described an attempt to treat chronic pain on an outpatient basis using a similar approach to those employed above with inpatients. In a pilot study they treated six patients in a three part management package. The first part involved symptom control with the use of relaxation, biofeedback, and autohypnosis. The second part involved stimulus control, taking a cognitive approach. This involves teaching the patient to identify those aspects of his thinking which are distorted and to delineate the underlying beliefs on which these are based. He is then helped to change his distorted thinking and personal beliefs using a form of Beck's cognitive therapy[46]. The object is to help the patient learn to reappraise reality and acquire a more appropriate view of the world. The third part of the treatment involves social system intervention. Essentially the family is instructed to reinforce non-pain behaviour so as to reduce secondary gain. The five patients who completed the treatment were followed-up at 6 months and 12 months. They showed a significant decrease in pain, hopelessness, depression and analgesic use. It was found that each part of the package made a contribution to the outcome.

Anderson et al.[47] reported a treatment programme for chronic pain which uses behaviour modification during a 7–8 week inpatient programme followed by 4 weeks on an outpatient basis. Their criteria for selection are stringent and patients involved in compensation cases are excluded as are those suffering from schizophrenia or severe personality disorders. No distinction is made between functional and organic pain. They report that 25 of 34 patients returned to full active lives and maintained this at follow-up from 6 months to 7 years later. The authors claim that the programme differs from others in that medication to relieve anxiety, depression and pain are gradually reduced, biofeedback and stimulators are not used and there is no group or individual psychiatric treatment. They ascribe the results to the behaviour modification approach. It is noteworthy, however, that work evaluation and counselling psychology is used in helping the patient to plan for the future.

Sarno[48] has reported on the results of treating chronic back pain in 28 patients. 19 improved to the point of normal or near normal activity, and at six months follow-up 18 had maintained their improvement. His multidisciplinary inpatient programme does not include operant conditioning. On theoretical grounds it has been decided that the secondary gains described by others are less important than the patient's intrapsychic conflicts, and accordingly, apart from physical treatments to restore muscle strength, all patients are treated with psychoanalytically orientated psychotherapy. Although Sarno suggests that the improvements achieved indicate that his theoretical stance is correct, he is well aware of the need to carry out a controlled study.

It can be seen that the multidisciplinary approach to the assessment and treatment of chronic pain is becoming increasingly common. In order to be successful, such programmes require a great deal of commitment from many departments within the general hospital[1]. Participants have to show a readiness to understand a wide range of models of pain and, in particular, to appreciate the contributions which can be made by other members of the team. Although these methods are time consuming, early results suggest that they may be cost-effective in reducing the amount of use which patients make of the health system as a whole.

ANTIDEPRESSANTS AND CHRONIC PAIN

Most patients with chronic pain are treated with antidepressants at some stage of their illness. Since it seems clear that the majority of patients with chronic pain do not suffer from a psychotic depressive syndrome which might be expected to respond to tricyclic medication, it has been suggested that these drugs may be acting in a somewhat different way when used for the treatment of intractable pain[49]. Recent studies suggest that the endogenous pain suppression system is to a considerable extent dependent upon brain concentrations of dopamine and serotonin. As Akil and Liebeskind[50] have shown these neurotransmitters appear to facilitate stimulation produced analgesia. These aspects of pain have been well reviewed by Liebeskind and Paul[51] and Kerr and Wilson[52].

Sternbach *et al.*[53] carried out a study aimed at demonstrating the effects on chronic pain, of altering brain serotonin activity. The patients were adult volunteers all of whom had organic pathology. Eleven patients were given reserpine for 3 days followed by placebos, five patients were given serotonin precursors followed by placebos, and nine patients were treated in a double-blind trial of chlorimipramine or amitriptyline and placebo. It was found that chlorimipramine decreased pain estimates to a significantly greater degree than placebo. Amitriptyline however, was no better than placebo. Reserpine did tend to increase pain and serotonin precursors reduced pain, but in neither instance was statistical significance achieved. Overall, this study supports the suggestion that serotonin levels are important in influencing the pain experience, but the evidence provided is not strong as might be expected with such small numbers of patients.

Kocher[54] has reported on the use of psychotropic drugs in treatment of chronic, severe pain associated with organic illness. He treated 103 inpatients with pain due to neurological and arthritic conditions which was resistant to conventional therapy. He used a number of drug combinations, including imipramine and levomepromazine, trimipramine and levomepromazine, imipramine and haloperidol and chlorimipramine and haloperidol. Of the 103 inpatients, 9 had no response, 60 had a fair to good response, and 32 had a very good response.

Bourhis *et al.*[55] reported on the treatment of pain in patients with cancer, using antidepressants and tranquillizers. They found that psychotropics were helpful but indicate that they acted not as analgesics but by reducing 'infirmity' and pain complaints. These authors believe that the use of narcotics in the treatment of cancer pain leads to its intractability. However, it seems equally plausible that it is the inappropriate use of narcotics which leads to problems, rather than their use as such. Bourhis *et al.*[55] maintains that 'what is important in considering chronic pain is above all the infirmity conferred upon the patient'.

Merskey and Hester[49] have reviewed their use of psychotropic drugs in 30 patients suffering severe chronic pain related to organic conditions such as postherpetic neuralgia, thalamic syndrome and carcinoma. They achieved moderately good results using a combination of phenothiazines, antidepressant drugs and antihistamines. Their findings suggest that these agents may alleviate pain by some action independent of their mood altering effects. However, since the pain experience encompasses an affective component it is difficult to draw distinctions of this sort.

HYPNOTHERAPY AND CHRONIC PAIN

Although its mechanism of action is not fully understood, hypnosis has long been known to influence the experience of pain[56, 57]. At present, however, it does not play a prominent part in the management of chronic pain; certainly there do not seem to be many reports from psychiatrists which indicate that they favour the regular use of hypnotherapy. There are a number of reasons for this situation. The proponents of hypnotherapy have over the years, tended to present their findings in a rather over enthusiastic and uncritical way. Too many claims were made for the treatment, which results in its indiscriminate use and inevitable disappointments as to its effectiveness. Two particular disadvantages are its variable effectiveness and the difficulty in predicting patient susceptibility. Furthermore, since a positive expectation on the patient's part is important to the success of the method, scepticism on the part of pain clinic staff can be an obstacle to its efficacy[58]. Since it is not easy to attain an uncritical acceptance of *any* treatment in most pain relief clinics (and especially those functioning in teaching hospitals committed to the scientific approach) it is not surprising that hypnotherapy plays such a relatively small part in their activities.

However, since a large part of the hypnotherapeutic effect may be ascribed to a non-specific reduction of anxiety, this can probably be achieved just as effectively by the use of somewhat more conventional psychological therapies. It should also be borne in mind that hypnotherapy functions best in patients with a relatively clearcut motivation to lose their pain. In many patients with chronic pain, psychodynamic factors may complicate the situation so that the patient is not motivated (at least unconsciously) to surrender his pain and sick-role status. As a consequence hypnotherapy is unlikely to be successful in their treatment. On the other hand, it clearly has a part to play in the management of pain where organic factors predominate and psychological factors are less prominent. Where it is effective, some patients can be taught to practice autohypnosis which affords them some control over their own pain problem.

OVERVIEW

There seems little doubt that the need for a multidisciplinary approach to the diagnosis and treatment of chronic pain is now generally accepted. The psychiatrist has become a key figure in the team and is expected to contribute to the detection of psychiatric syndromes as well as the delineation of the psychodynamics operating in individual patients and their families. It is now necessary to determine which forms of treatment are most effective in managing pain, so that where possible, the most cost-effective method may be used. It is also important to develop skills and techniques for the early recognition of pain syndromes in which psychosocial factors play a prominent role, so that appropriate management may be instituted and unnecessary investigations and treatments avoided.

References

1 Pilowsky, I. (1976). The psychiatrist and the pain clinic. *Am. J. Psychiatry*, **133**, 752

2 Morgan, C. D., Kremer, E. and Gaylor, M. (1979). The behavioural medicine unit: A new facility. *Compre Psychiatry*, **20**, 29

3a Pilowsky, I. (1969). Abnormal illness behaviour. *Br. J. Med. Psychol.*, **42**, 347

3b Pilowsky, I. (1971). The diagnosis of abnormal illness behaviour. *Aust. N. Z. J. Psychiatry*, **5**, 136

3c Pilowsky, I. (1978). A general classification of abnormal illness behaviours. *Br. J. Med. Psychol.*, **51**, 131

4 Merskey, H. (1979). Psychological aspects of pain relief. In Swerdlow, M. (ed.) *Relief of Intractable Pain*. 2nd edn. pp. 21–48 (Amsterdam: Excerpta Medica)

5 Mechanic, D. and Vokart, E. H. (1966). Stress, illness behaviour and the sick role. *Am. Sociol. Rev.*, **26**, 51

6 Pilowsky, I. (1967). Dimensions of hypochondriasis. *Br. J. Psychiatry*, **113**, 89

7 Cowden, R. C. and Brown, J. E. (1956). The use of a physical symptom as a defence against psychosis. *J. Abnorm. Soc. Psychol.*, **53**, 133

8 Pilowsky, I. and Spence, N. D. (1976). Illness behaviour syndromes associated with intractable pain. *Pain*, **2**, 61

9 Pilowsky, I. and Spence, N. D. (1975). Patterns of illness behaviour in patients with intractable pain. *Pain*, **19**, 279

10 Pilowsky, I., Chapman, C. R. and Bonica, J. J. (1977). Pain, depression and illness behaviour in a pain clinic population. *Pain*, **4**, 183

11 Pilowsky, I. (1978). Psychodynamic aspects of pain experience. In Sternbach, R. A. (ed.). *The Psychology of Pain*, pp. 203–217. (New York: Raven Press)

12. Wall, P. D. (1979). On the relation of injury to pain. *Pain*, **6**, 253

13 Engel, G. (1959). Psychogenic pain and the pain-prone patient. *Am. J. Med.*, **26**, 899

14 Bursten, B. and D'Esopo, R. (1965). The obligation to remain sick. *Arch. Gen. Psychiatry*, **12**, 402

15 Woodforde, J. M. and Merskey, H. (1972). Personality traits of patients with chronic pain. *J. Psychosom. Res.*, **16**, 167

16 Merskey, H. (1972). Personality traits of psychiatric patients with chronic pain. *J. Psychosom. Res.*, **16**, 163

17 Bond, M. R. (1976). Pain and personality in cancer patients. In Bonica, J. J. and Albe-Fessard, D. (eds.) *Advances in Pain Research and Therapy*, 1, pp. 311–316. (New York: Raven Press)

18 Sternbach, R. A., Murphy, R. W., Akeson, W. H. and Wolf, S. R. (1973). Chronic low-back pain – the low-back loser. *Postgrad. Med.*, **53**, 135

19 Gentry, W. D., Shows, W. D. and Thomas, M. (1974). Chronic low back pain: A psychological profile. *Psychosomatics*, **15**, 174

20 McCreary, C., Turner, J. and Dawson, E. (1977). Differences between functional versus organic low back pain patients. *Pain*, **4**, 73

21 Leavitt, F., Garron, D. C., D'Angelo, C. M. and McNiell, T. W. (1979). Low back pain in patients with and without demonstrable organic disease. *Pain*, **6**, 191

22 Blumetti, A. E. and Modesti, L. M. (1976). Psychological predictors of success or failure of surgical intervention for intractable back pain. In Bonica, J. J. and Albe-Fessard, D. (eds.). *Advances in Pain Research and Therapy*, 1, pp. 323–325. (New York: Raven Press)

23 Spring, A. Wittek, R. and Worz, R. (1976). Interdependence of low back pain and psychiatric symptomatology. In Bonica, J. J. and Albe-Fessard, D. (eds.). *Advances in Pain Research and Therapy*, 1, pp. 943–947. (New York: Raven Press)

24 Lloyd, G. G., Wolkind, S. N., Greenwood, R. and Harris, D. J. (1979). A psychiatric study of patients with persistent low back pain. *Rheumatol. Rehabil.*, **18**, 30

25 Gross, S. M. and Vacchiano, R. B. (1973). Personality correlates of patients with temperomandibular joint dysfunction. *J. Prosthet. Dent.,* **30,** 326

26 Lupton, D. E. (1969). Psychological aspects of temperomandibular joint dysfunction. *J. Am. Dent. Assoc.,* **79,** 131

27 Delaney, J. F. (1976). Atypical facial pain as a defense against psychosis. *Am. J. Psychiatry,* **133,** 1151

28 Schoenberg, B., Carr, A. C., Kutscher, A. H. and Zegarelli, E. V. (1971). Chronic idiopathic orolingual pain: Psychogenesis of burning mouth. *N.Y. State J. Med.,* **71,** 1832

29 Moldofsky, H., Scarisbrick, P., England, R. and Smythe, H. (1975). Musculoskeletal symptoms and non-REM sleep disturbance in patients with 'fibrositis syndrome' and healthy subjects. *Psychosom. Med.,* **37,** 341

30 Moldofsky, H. and Walsh, J. J. (1978). Plasma tryptophan and musculoskeletal pain in non-articular rheumatism ('fibrositis syndrome'). *Pain,* **5,** 65

31 Vaughn, R., Pall, M. L. and Haynes, S. N. (1977). Frontalis EMG response to stress in subjects with frequent muscle contraction headaches. *Headache,* **16,** 313

32 van Boxtel, A., Roozeveld van der ven, J. (1978). Differential EMG activity in subjects with contraction headaches related to mental effort. *Headache,* **17,** 233

33 Delaplane, R., Ifabuminyi, O. I., Merskey, H. and Zarfas, J. (1978). Significance of pain in psychiatric hospital patients. *Pain,* **4,** 361

34 Merskey, H. and Boyd, D. (1978). Emotional adjustment and chronic pain, *Pain,* **5,** 173

35 Mohamed, S. N., Weisz, G. M. and Waring, E. M. (1978). The relationship of chronic pain to depression, marital adjustment and family dynamics. *Pain,* **5,** 285

36 Chapman, C. R., Sola, A. E. and Bonica, J. J. (1979). Illness behaviour and depression compared in pain center and private practice patients. *Pain,* **6,** 1

37 Cairns, D., Thomas, L., Mooney, V. and Pace, J. B. (1976). A comprehensive treatment approach to chronic low back pain. *Pain,* **2,** 301

38 Fordyce, W. E. (1976). *Behavioural Methods in Chronic Pain and Illness.* (St. Louis: C. V. Mosby)

39 Ignelzi, R. J., Sternbach, R. A. and Timmermans, G. (1977). The pain ward follow-up analyses. *Pain,* **3,** 227

40 Newman, R. L., Seres, J. L., Jspe, L. P. and Carlington, B. (1978). Multidisciplinary treatment of chronic pain: Long term follow-up of low back pain patients. *Pain,* **4,** 283

41 Newman, R. I., Painter, J. R. and Seres, J. L. (1978). A therapeutic milieu for chronic pain patients. *J. Human Stress,* **4,** 8

42 Swanson, D. W., Maruta, T. and Swenson, W. M. (1979). Results of behaviour modification in treatment of chronic pain. *Psychosom. Med.,* **41,** 55

43 Swanson, D. W., Swenson, W. M., Maruta, T. and Floreen, H. C. (1978). The dissatisfied patient with chronic pain. *Pain,* **4,** 367

44 Maruta, T., Swanson, D. W., Finlayson, R. E. (1979). Drug abuse and dependency in patients with chronic pain. *Mayo Clin. Proc.,* **54,** 241

45 Katami, M. and Rush, A. J. (1978). A pilot study of the treatment of outpatients with chronic pain: Symptom control, stimulus control and social system intervention. *Pain,* **5,** 163

46 Beck, A. T. (1974). The development of depression: A cognitive model. In Friedman, R. J. and Katz, M. M. (eds.). *The Psychology of Depression.* (New York: Wiley)

47 Anderson, T. P., Cole, T. M., Gullickson, G., Hudgens, A. and Roberts, A. H. (1977). Behaviour modification of chronic pain. *Clin. Orthop.,* **129,** 96

48 Sarno, J. E. (1976). Chronic back pain and psychic conflict. *Scand. J. Rehab. Med.,* **8,** 143

49 Merskey, H. and Hester, R. A. (1972). The treatment of chronic pain with psychotropic drugs. *Postgrad. Med.,* **48,** 594

50 Akil, H. and Liebeskind, J. C. (1975). Monoaminergic mechanisms of stimulation produced analgesia. *Brain Res.,* **94,** 279

51 Liebeskind, J. C. and Paul, L. A. (1977). Psychological and physiological mechanisms of pain. *Ann. Rev. Psychol.,* **28,** 41

52 Kerr, F. W. L. and Wilson, P. R. (1978). Pain. *Ann. Rev. Neurosci.,* **1,** 83

53 Sternbach, R. A., Janowsky, D. S., Huey., L. Y. and Segal, D. S. (1976). Effects of altering brain serotonin activity on human chronic pain. In Bonica, J. J. and Albe-Fessard, D. (eds.). *Advances in Pain Research and Therapy,* 1, pp. 601–606. (New York: Raven Press)

54 Kocher, R. (1976). Use of psychotropic drugs for the treatment of chronic severe pain. In Bonica, J. J. and Albe-Fessard, D. (eds.). *Advances in Pain Research and Therapy,* 1, pp. 579–582. (New York: Raven Press)

55. Bourhis, A., Boudouresque, G., Pellet, W., Fondarai, J., Ponzio, J. and Spitalier, J. M. (1978). Pain infirmity and psychotropic drugs in oncology. *Pain.* **4,** 263

56 Hilgard, E. R. (1978). Hypnosis and pain. In Sternbach, R. A. (ed.). *The Psychology of Pain,* pp. 219–240. (New York: Raven Press)

57 Crasilneck, H. B. and Hall, J. A. (1973). Clinical hypnosis in problems of pain. *Am. J. Clin. Hypnosis,* **15,** 153

58 Finer, B. (1979). Hypnotherapy in pain of advanced cancer. In Bonica, J. J. and Ventafridda, V. (eds.). *Advances in Pain Research and Therapy.* pp. 223–29 (New York: Raven Press)

3

Current views on the management of a pain relief centre

S. Lipton

INTRODUCTION

Old ideas die hard and the biblical feeling that original sin had to be expiated by human suffering is still present today. Thus it is only in the last few decades that any thought has been given to the alleviation of chronic pain in a scientific fashion[1-4]. If the cause of the pain was unknown, or was untreatable, or if the normal treatment failed, then very little was offered to the sufferers, except perhaps opiate drugs. The idea that the pain in these cases had become a disease and this disease needed treatment was a strange one. The wonders and cures of medicine and surgery during the last fifty years seemed to blind everyone, except a few pioneers, to the basic thought that medicine originated in the relief of pain and suffering and should progress in that direction also for the relief of chronic pain and the suffering due to it. The causes of pain are legion, and pain relief clinics have arisen to devote themselves to chronic, i.e. intractable long-term pain; there is some modern thought that a lead in the treatment of acute pain might be given also[5].

The amount of existing pain is enormous and unbelievable until one tries to quantify it. For instance, in considering cancer pain, recognition must be given to the fact that one out of every five people will die from cancer and that about 70% of these will die in some degree of pain if untreated[6,7]. Thus approximately 14% of people dying will die in pain from cancer. Non-malignant conditions also cause chronic pain and are equally widespread in the population and exist over a longer time scale. Because there are official figures available on the amount of sickness and absence from work, an assessment of the frequency of some painful chronic conditions and their effect can be made[8]. Back pain is such a one. In 1975 in

61

the United Kingdom, there were 391000 spells of loss of work and 13.2 million days lost due to back pain[9].

The cost due to back pain from loss of production to industry and to the gross national product is enormous. The pain and suffering both physically and financially on a personal basis is also great. This is a condition which occurs frequently, yet few people are incapacitated permanently by it. It is estimated that in America its cost to the community is $12 billion each year[8]. This is the bill for only one chronic painful condition. There are many others and the hospitalization and prescribing for them, and the self-medications bought over the counter, are an enormous drain on the productivity and wealth of a country.

The organized treatment of chronic pain in Western countries and in Japan has evolved by the gradual development of pain relief centres, where the central aim is not so much the management of pain as the treatment of it. Naturally, in those unfortunate patients whose pain cannot be entirely relieved, it must be managed in the best way possible. Pain relief centres are of differing complexity both in organization and in the treatments they offer. The problems of organizing and managing a pain relief centre will be dealt with under the following headings:

1. Functions of a pain relief centre
   (A) Diagnosis
   (B) Treatment
   (C) Teaching
   (D) Research
   (E) Service to other departments

2. The scope of a pain relief centre
   (A) Types
   (B) Limitations
   (C) Special Units

3. Organization of a pain relief centre
   (A) Staff arrangements
   (B) Patient arrangements
   (C) Additional facilities

4. Management of a pain relief centre
   (A) Techniques

(B) Growth of the clinic

(C) Medico-legal problems

FUNCTIONS OF A PAIN RELIEF CENTRE

(A) Diagnosis

A major purpose of any pain relief centre is to diagnose the cause of the pain in those patients referred to it. This may sound a truism but it is remarkable how often a patient is referred for treatment with only the vaguest of, or an absence of, a diagnosis. As in all other branches of medicine, the first necessity of treatment is to know what is being treated and this means diagnosis. All the arrangements of the pain relief centre are organized to this purpose and only afterwards the treatment. Of course in some cases a diagnosis is impossible, but before treatment is undertaken in such patients on an empirical basis, the lack of a diagnosis must be faced by the pain relief centre team.

It will also follow that a particular clinician must not give opinions outside his or her specialty until the necessary expertise is acquired. This means that some members of the team, such as the anaesthetist, who is especially well equipped to deal with needle techniques of pain relief, will have to undergo a conscious development of clinical skills which have been overshadowed in his normal practice. A neurosurgeon giving an opinion on a chest would be a corresponding example.

(B) Treatment

Since the treatment of pain will involve the treatment of any portion of the body, it follows that comprehensive treatment cannot be provided by one clinician. This is why the most modern centres are large multidisciplinary ones, where numbers of different specialists are brought together so that their individual skills in diagnosis and treatment summate into a larger whole. Thus the patient obtains the best possible treatment available. This can be of any type such as medical, surgical, psychiatric, orthopaedic or other. The methods in which these specialists, who form the pain relief centre team, are organized and managed and the scope of their work is discussed in later sections, but, just as clinicians of one specialty should be careful in their diagnosis, so they must also be careful in their treatment. There can be overlapping of treatment by members of the team but the most valuable and economical use of the skills occurs when each tends to do those things for which he or she was trained. This does not mean that a special skill cannot be acquired by suitable learning. This leads on to the question of teaching.

(C) Teaching

This is of much wider scope than suggested at the end of the previous paragraph as it is axiomatic that any medical group should try to advance the state of their art. This means informing other doctors and nurses of their results, of the effects of new drugs and of new methods. This immediately requires that proper records be kept and statistics worked out. Opinions as to the value of particular methods and drugs are important but they cannot take the place of proper records and satisfactory statistics.

When the pain relief centre hospital is part of a medical school, then teaching will automatically be part of its function. When it is not physically in a teaching centre, medical students may well visit it, but in any case it must train its own staff, both nursing and medical. Orientation lectures and specific training need to be carried out, and these are geared on the one hand to nurses and doctors spending a short time (say two weeks to two months) at the centre, while those requiring a more comprehensive training stay for longer periods. Thus students and residents (nurses or doctors) will require broadly based training to familiarize themselves with basic techniques and broad varieties of intractable pain and its treatment.

Senior residents and visiting specialists will require more concentrated and detailed information and proper training programmes must be worked out. Finally, there must be a full training programme for those doctors, resident or visitors, who wish to develop expertise in pain relief practice so that they may take up this work when properly trained.

Also, under the heading of 'Teaching' comes the question of information. The centre should provide information, indeed 'propaganda', to its local population and the population in general, to doctors in the surrounding area and to local and central government. This should be considered as one of the most important sections of the work that the centre can carry out. The information should not only be on what the centre itself can carry out, but should be preventative as well; for instance much back pain could be prevented if people would learn how to lift heavy objects properly.

(D) Research

This subject naturally falls under several headings:

(a) Epidemiology

One of the great handicaps to people working in the pain relief field is that there is little knowledge of the relationship and frequency of pain to the general population and to specific groups of the population. A little of this information is available such as the incidence of back pain in some industrial groups[9], but the gaps are very wide indeed. Further, there is little known about the self-cure rate and whether this is affected by treatment. If continuous and full statistics are kept of the pain clinic patients, then in due course some of these questions will be answered.

(b) Drugs

There are now available drugs of the agonist–antagonist variety such as Temgesic (buprenorphine) and Fortral (pentazocine), non-narcotic drugs such as Acupan (nefopam), and other varieties of drugs or modifications of old ones, such as Dolobid (diflunisal), which have been released for general use. It will be necessary for the pain relief centre to use these drugs where indicated and to assess them in the field. Often drugs are released for general use and the problems and difficulties in their use only found after prolonged use and prescribing. Not only is it necessary to examine the new drugs, but to use the older ones satisfactorily and properly[10] and schemes of research should reflect this. A clinical pharmacologist is invaluable in this type of research.

(c) Evaluation of new techniques

New techniques for pain relief are constantly being devised and details published. Any large pain relief centre must keep up to date on these but the original papers on them cannot be accepted blindly so a scheme of clinical appraisal of such new techniques must be carried out. The results of such evaluations must be published with such modifications as have been added. For instance, such techniques as epidural morphine and subarachnoid morphine[11] have recently been introduced. Transcutaneous external neural stimulation[12,13] for post-operative pain is a little less recent. Acupuncture[13], alpha feedback and hypnosis[14] are all subjects on which further research information is desired. Not only must new techniques be evaluated but also new methods of using older techniques.

(d) Evaluation of new equipment

As with (c) above this type of assessment is absolutely essential. Often a piece of new equipment is used for an old purpose and then a scientific investigation takes place as to whether it has any advantages, whether it is safe to patient and staff, and whether it is safe in special places, say in the operating theatre near piped gases.

(e) Projects
These will be the special research projects carried out by the personnel of the pain relief centre. Projects of this type are most essential to the growth and standing of the centre and should be of both short and long term. All trainees should be encouraged to take part in such projects and to initiate and complete one if their period in the pain relief centre is long enough.

(f) Publication
All staff are encouraged to publish. Negative as well as positive papers must be written. A definite arrangement must be made so that advice on writing for publication can be obtained from experienced members of the pain relief team.

(g) Funding
Research projects may be funded specially by local, university or national research bodies, or may be carried out by the internal arrangements of the pain relief centre. While much funding of research projects occurs from within the pain relief centre, any major funds for special equipment or prolonged projects will usually have to be obtained from outside bodies. This necessitates applications for such funds and the writing of these applications is a very specialized field. Undoubtedly, there will be one or more members of team who are expert in this field and it is most important they help those not as experienced.

(E) Service to other departments
The most important function of a pain relief centre is to deal with its own patients, but it may, because of the special techniques available to it, become a diagnostic and to a lesser extent a treatment centre for other specialties. For instance, most pain relief centres will use the technique of lumbar sympathetic block as a treatment for causalgic pain. In the centre itself, this technique is used as a diagnostic measure to see whether those patients who have a causalgic element to their pain (shown by dysaesthesia, or a sensation of heat in their pain) will respond to a lumbar sympathetic block. It may well be that vascular surgeons wish to use the expertise of the centre by referring some of their patients with abnormalities of the vascular tree in the lower limb, to see if a diagnostic lum-

bar sympathetic block will show benefit to the patient, either from the point of view of relief of pain or by an increased blood supply increasing the claudication walking distance[15]. Likewise, from a treatment point of view many orthopaedic departments request that an epidural steroid injection be carried out by the pain relief centre as a service. In general terms the use of the pain relief centre facilities by other clinicians is to be encouraged, but the size and scope of this use must be quantified so that the centre can be adequately staffed. If the staffing is limited, then certain categories of work will have to be refused. However, ways can be found around this difficulty by training somebody from the referring specialty in the technique required (see p. 70).

THE SCOPE OF A PAIN RELIEF CLINIC

(A) Types

There is considerable literature[3,8,16-19] on the various types of pain relief clinic. One type of pain clinic merges into another but there are certainly two extreme basic types. The first is the simplest where a single doctor sees a small number of patients suffering from chronic pain problems. The facilities available are of the simplest and the scope of this type of clinic accordingly abbreviated. It will consist of one doctor, of any discipline but often an anaesthetist, examining patients and treating them by simple means such as diagnostic and neurolytic blocks.

At the opposite end of the scale of types is the clinic where there is a large team of doctors all interested in relieving chronic pain, working together by pooling their knowledge and resources. This is known as the multidisciplinary pain relief centre. It will have available beds, nurses, outpatient and inpatient facilities, ancillary staff, the use of all the special facilities in the hospital; it can call on other specialist medical staff if necessary. In particular, there is no type of pain relief technique that is not available to it, and it will carry out all the functions mentioned. The number of large pain relief clinics is steadily rising with the United States of America having about twice as many as the rest of the world[18].

As might be expected, most pain relief clinics are neither as small as the simple type nor as large as the multidisciplinary type, but lie midway between the two in size and development. In this third group a few doctors, usually around three, will have most of the hospital facilities that the multidisciplinary type has but because of limitations of time and space may not carry out some of the longer and more complicated procedures.

There is a great variation between clinics of this intermediate type. Some of them are as large as the multidisciplinary type but the team prefers the more informal working of the intermediate system. There is in fact a basic difference between the two. Many patients attending a pain relief clinic have relatively simple problems which are soon dealt with, but when this does not happen arrangements are made in a multidisciplinary clinic for the team of specialists or five or more of them to see the patient together. So that a physician, surgeon, anaesthetist, orthopaedic surgeon, neurologist, and psychiatrist, may do this. In the intermediate type, it is only on very special occasions that a joint opinion of this type is obtained; more usually the normal procedures of referral through the outpatient clinics are used. These are organized so that an opinion can be obtained either the same day or the following day. The advantage of the combined multidisciplinary approach is that the very best opinion on the condition and its treatment can be provided but this is at the expense of two-thirds of the team present who contribute nothing. It is a very effective method of combating future accusations of misdiagnosis and mistreatment and problems in regard to malpractice litigation have to be considered in some countries. Where this is not a feature a much more effective use of team members' time can be made in the 'intermediate' type of clinic. It must be remembered that the considerations about pain relief clinics in this chapter are being looked at from a European and specifically British angle, and therefore allowance must be made for this. It is axiomatic that all the ideas in this chapter will need modification before being used in another country.

(B) Limitations

It will be obvious that only the largest pain relief centres can encompass all functions and that in most cases the centre has limitations imposed on it. These limitations depend on:

(a) Choice of patient

The particular patients to be seen decide the scope of the individual pain relief clinic. A pilot study of chronic pain patients may be necessary to show this either in an established clinic to show if its arrangements are correct or before a new one is commissioned to check the type of case it will receive. At the Centre for Pain Relief in Walton Hospital, Liverpool, nearly 30% of patients treated have inoperable cancer, while in two other British clinics[18] cancer pain accounts for only 15% and 17% respectively of the patients seen. For low back pain the figures in these three clinics are 25%, 22%, 21%.

The clinic can either be an open clinic, in other words a clinic to which all doctors in or out of the hospital can refer patients, or it can be an internal clinic when only the doctors in the hospital where the centre is based can refer patients. Facilities of the internal clinic can be extended to doctors in other hospitals. When a patient is referred from outside the centre, the patient has to be dealt with *ab initio*, but when the patient is admitted from a hospital clinic, to a large extent the write-up and the initial work-up of the patient have been carried out. In fact, this preliminary work-up can be made a condition of admittance. More time and a larger staff is necessary if an open centre policy is adopted.

(b) Inpatient facilities

Depending on whether the pain clinic is simple, intermediate or multi-disciplinary, the inpatient facilities will range from none to fully adequate. Conversely, there is no point in setting up an intermediate or multidisciplinary pain relief clinic unless inpatient facilities are provided. Further note must be taken of exactly what facilities are offered or available. For instance, if a pain relief clinic has ten inpatient beds in ten different wards, it would change immediately the scope of the work possible compared to having them in the same or two adjacent wards.

(c) The staff available

Here again the scope of the pain relief clinic is closely controlled by numbers of nurses, the time(s) at which the operating theatre is available and whether an image intensifier is available. There is no need to enumerate all the difficulties possible but one must be mentioned here in relation to hospital beds. When inpatients are treated who provides the medical cover for them? Who acts as houseman or registrar? If, to continue the previous idea, there are ten patients in ten different wards, who looks after them? Questions such as these must be solved by the pain team.

(d) Techniques

The techniques of pain relief used are dependent on the expertise and preferences of the specialist members of the team. A decision on the types of pain treated and who amongst the specialist members of the team will take responsibility for each must be decided by discussion of the whole team. Sometimes there are two ways of tackling a particular technique because the training of one specialist enables him to become adept at needle techniques for example while another operates surgically.

A simple example can be given. The open cordotomy carried out by surgical means is performed by neurosurgeons. This holds good throughout the world. However, the modern method of percutaneous cervical cordotomy is carried out through an 18 gauge spinal needle placed in the lateral cervical C_1–C_2 region. It is a straightforward procedure provided the special equipment is available and the doctor performing the technique is properly trained[20]. In most countries of the world this technique is carried out by neurosurgeons also, but in some places, the British Isles being an obvious example, it is carried out by specialists other than neurosurgeons, mainly by anaesthesiologists. The reason for this is that in the British Isles, neurosurgeons are extremely busy and there is no dearth of other neurosurgical problems and work. Usually in pain relief centres carrying out the percutaneous cervical cordotomy the anaesthesiologist and neurosurgeon work closely together with a neurologist and radiologist, and problems such as this are easily sorted out. However, it must be borne in mind that the common usage of the country involved is best followed when it comes to organizing a centre.

There is one great advantage in having a certain amount of overlap in the abilities of the different members of the team since, inevitably, cover is needed for holiday leave or when somebody becomes ill. The pain clinic runs more smoothly if one of its members can partially deputize for another; this is not a replacement policy, it is merely a question of helping out.

Another example would be the decision on the best way the psychiatric member of the team is going to fit in. There is no doubt that psychiatric help has an enormous place in pain relief. A large proportion of patients with psychiatric problems have pain as well, while patients in chronic pain develop neuroses, and therefore the presence of a psychiatrist as a member of the pain relief team is exceedingly valuable[21]. The presence should be an active one, with the psychiatrist seeing his own referrals and those from other members of the team. It is important that a decision is made on whether all patients should have a psychiatric assessment or only some of them. The psychiatrist member will take the lead here. (see Chapter 2). When all active treatment has failed, the only method remaining to help the patient may be to alter the patient's attitude to his pain.

(e) Clerical staff
Clerical staff are required in larger numbers than would be thought. Apart from typists, admission, ward and filing clerks who must be available as

in any hospital department. Some thought has to be given to this section of the staff in relation to who arranges follow-up visits decided on by medical staff, who compiles and distributes operations lists, are clinic, ward and operation notes to be typed, are record clerks to be employed and how many? Decisions must also be made on computer filing for research purposes, and on how many extra clerical staff are necessary to cover the research undertaken. In other words, if this particular section of staff is short in number it produces limitations on all other forms of activity and may curtail some of them completely.

(f) The appointments system
No appointments system works perfectly so care must be taken with this key section of activity. If the allowance of time for patients in the out-patient department is too short, the waiting room fills up; if too long, highly trained people are inactive and expensive ancillary medical and nursing time is wasted. There must be some previous thought on who deals with the patient who arrives late through no fault of his own, even if the decision is that there is no one to deal with this patient and he must be given another appointment or offered an overnight stay so he can be seen the following day. Again, some patients arrive on the wrong day, or a physician requests an urgent consultation in the middle of an already overflowing clinic. Consultations referred from one member of the pain relief team to another must also be allowed for as must a complication of a routine nerve block occurring in the middle of a clinic. These problems are to some extent dealt with in organization, but unless allowance is made for such happenings there will be very definite limitations placed on the working of the clinic.

(C) Special units
Chronic pain of limited type is sometimes treated in special units equipped to deal with one or a few types of pain. This may be because of staffing difficulties, the particular interests of the doctor involved, or through potential malpractice litigation. These smaller more specialized units for pain relief arise in part because multidisciplinary pain relief clinics are becoming larger and larger with increasing staff and complicated organization. The probability is that these units, whether inside or out-side the hospital, will not be part of the pain relief clinic, although any help or advice in respect of pain relief will be readily given to them. Only the largest of multidisciplinary pain relief clinics will be able to provide help to these various clinics and a sense of proportion needs to be kept on

what it is possible for the pain relief clinic to undertake and what it should commit itself to. Discussion on this point will be necessary between the pain relief clinic team members. These *specialized units* may be actual clinics or provide services only. They may, for instance, deal with:

Back pain

In this type of specialized clinic some of the ordinary diagnostic blocking services of the pain relief clinic are available and also special techniques such as facet blocks and facet nerve coagulations[22].

Migraine

Most migraine is of a temporary nature and is controlled by well known therapy. However, some patients do have migraine of extremely severe and almost continuous type. These patients should be investigated and treated initially by the neurological member of the pain team. If their severe headaches persist it may be useful for them to attend a migraine clinic specifically orientated to this type of problem where they can get urgent treatment and help during and in between severe bouts.

Acupuncture

This is a complete subject on its own, but, with the understanding of the physiological action of acupuncture by stimulating endogenous opiate production, its use in pain relief is acknowledged[23]. The author is extremely wary of those doctors who believe acupuncture can treat any condition and use it for such purposes. It is known to be a useful agent for pain relief.

Relaxation

Here the emphasis is on relaxation either by hypnosis, simple relaxation techniques, or other methods[13,14].

Biofeedback

This is an established procedure for relaxing patients where spasm is a feature. For instance patients, who by habit or because of their work keep their heads still, tend to get stiffness of the muscles of the neck and scalp and will develop pain in the muscles attached to the scalp aponeurosis. By using an electromyograph the activity of these muscles can be shown to the patient on a dial or as an intensity of light. The patient can then develop the ability to control the tension through learning to control the movement of the indicator on the dial or the intensity of the light. After a time, such control becomes automatic and the apparatus is not necessary[13].

Operant conditioning
This is a psychological method of altering the patient's behaviour to pain in that although he cannot be relieved of his pain, he is taught to live with it and carry on as normal a life as possible despite pain[24].

Counselling
This sounds a very simple and innocuous method of treating a patient with pain but very often the patients have never really considered how they can change their pain themselves by altering their lifestyle. Thus the specialist giving the counselling for pain will need to be as expert in this field as say a psychiatrist giving treatment for neurosis or psychosis. Often this type of counselling is conducted through the psychiatric or psychological department and must be regarded as a very special expert procedure. As a simple example, a patient who has chronic back pain may have an unsuitable job which entails stooping and lifting. The patient may never have considered altering his job and this must be brought to his attention. However, the patient may know that it is this work that causes the problem and yet will not consider change. The counsellor then has the difficult task of finding out why the patient has embarked on such a self-destructive process and endeavours to correct the situation.

ORGANIZATION OF A PAIN RELIEF CLINIC

(A) Staff arrangements

(a) The team
The basic structure of a larger pain relief clinic is to have a team of different specialists working together and using their combined expertise and knowledge to relieve the chronic painful conditions of those patients presenting to the clinic. In a multidisciplinary clinic, a number of specialists see each pain problem together, though usually there is a primary physician, often one of the multidisciplinary team, to screen new patients. Many clinics arrange for the history and preliminary examination to be carried out by a person other than the physician or specialist who will be in charge of that patient. This saves a certain amount of time

and allows the specialist to see more patients. This system is a useful arrangement for training purposes.

The specialists normally available are a physician, a surgeon, orthopaedic surgeon, neurologist, an anaesthetist, neurosurgeon and psychiatrist. This panel of specialists is not meant to be fixed and is dependent upon the availability of such specialists. In general terms, the idea that all specialists see every patient no longer finds favour in the setting up of new clinics and the re-organization of established ones. The reasons are straightforward – there is far more work available for all these specialists than they can conveniently manage. To have six of them say, examining one patient is excellent theoretically, but it means that four of them at least will have very little to contribute. It may be interesting for the physicians themselves, and can be adopted as a teaching measure, but as a routine method of treatment it leaves much to be desired. A consensus seems to be arising that one specialist of any discipline should see the patient initially and take responsibility for him. Any investigations, whether biochemical, radiological or other, are carried out and the patient is then reviewed. If the patient comes from a distance, this is done as quickly as possible and the patient may be kept in the hospital as an inpatient if ill enough, or may reside near the hospital while a decision is being made. The primary physician re-assesses the patient, decides if a decision on treatment can be made, and if so arranges this. If not, a decision is made as to which other specialist is required to give an opinion and help, and this consultation is arranged. In most cases in large centres this can be done within 48 hours, often almost immediately, as the second opinion specialist works in the same hospital. A decision can then be made on further treatment and this is conveyed to the referring doctor if necessary, or arrangements are made to carry out any special investigations or treatment. If a decision is made that treatment is to be say by psychiatric or orthopaedic means, then the patient is referred to the relevant member of the team.

(b) The chain of command

It is axiomatic that one of the physicians of the pain team has to take administrative charge of the whole centre; in a larger clinic it is helpful to have a 'deputy' when the director is away for any reason. It is important also that a primary physician keeps contact with each patient's progress. It is this primary physician whom the patient can regard as 'my doctor'. It is this physician who decides initial treatment, diagnosis, and disposal, and who keeps in touch with the referring physician relaying the patient's progress. It is this physician who monitors the patient's progress when referred to other departments and makes sure that proper follow-up has been arranged and details sent to the referring physician. The arrangements made for the follow-up of these patients is usually by them re-visiting the clinic, but in special cases, the follow-up can be effected by telephone. Decisions on these points depend on the patient's mobility, how far he lives from the clinic, the expected time scale of initiated treatment, the possibility of complications and finally whether or not he will be 'put up to' the full multidisciplinary panel. The primary physician will ensure that the patient has been properly worked up for this panel and will present the case, the problem and all the medical evidence and investigations. He will also ensure that the panel's opinions and suggestions are carried out and inform the referring physician (and the patient) about this. Most pain relief clinics have certain well defined methods of referring certain types of patients to particular members of the pain panel or to particular sections of the clinic. This aspect will be defined later.

(c) The small clinic
The pain relief centres mentioned so far are large organizations with many staff of all types and with the access to all departments of the hospital. The largest number of multidisciplinary clinics is to be found in the USA[18]; in the United Kingdom and other parts of the world there are relatively few pain relief clinics of this complexity, the majority being quite small, depending on one physician, usually an anaesthetist, interested in pain relief. Most pain relief clinics in the past originated in this fashion. They start with no fixed facilities, making the best use of space and time not allocated to other disciplines. If no inpatient facilities are possible, then only measures which do not require hospitalization (such as straightforward diagnosis, blocks, TNS, acupuncture, and drug therapy) are used. As the clinic develops, then other facilities are added. The use of inpatient beds in conjunction with the availability of an image intensifier X-ray is a tremendous step forward. Gradually the small clinic becomes an intermediate type clinic and growth continues.

(d) Suggestions
The problem of staffing pain relief clinics properly is one which has exercised the minds of all the specialties involved in pain relief work. With regard to the anaesthetist member of the team, the Association of Anaesthetists of Great Britain and Ireland set up a subcommittee to study

this problem. Their recommendations were that each hospital dealing with a population of about two hundred and fifty thousand should have one anaesthesia specialist who was prepared to spend two sessions (half days) per week on pain relief work. This particular specialist would be carrying out the simpler methods of pain relief and control and would not perform such procedures as percutaneous cervical cordotomy or pituitary injection of alcohol. However, coeliac plexus block, lumbar sympathetic block, phenol injections, and other therapeutic or diagnostic blocks would come within his scope. In each larger hospital catering for a population of about one million or more, usually including a neurosurgical or neurological department, there should be two anaesthetists in the pain team who between them provide eleven sessions per week, that is one whole week's work. Each of them would supply half a week's work and in this way holiday and emergency cover could be provided. The pain relief team at these base hospitals would be able to offer a pain relieving service of a fairly complete nature. They would provide all the usual pain relieving techniques, including percutaneous cervical cordotomy, pituitary injection of alcohol, dorsal column stimulation, and even cerebral stimulation.

(B) Patient arrangements

(a) Allocation
Each pain relief clinic has its own particular method of allocating the new patients to members of the multidisciplinary team. This system must be kept simple, one suggestion[24] being that, for the initial consultation:

(1) Head and neck pain is referred to the neurologist member of the team.
(2) Central pain to the neurosurgeon.
(3) Back pain to the orthopaedic surgeon.
(4) Neurosis and psychosis to the psychiatrist.
(5) Rheumatoid arthritis pain to a rheumatologist.
(6) All other types of pain to the anaesthetist.

The members of the team must decide on the system by mutual accord and obviously it will vary depending on the available specialists. One of the problems associated with allocating patients in this way is that the patient may not improve and yet continues to be seen as an outpatient without any real change in his pain. A multidisciplinary clinic has the facilities to avoid this by presenting the patient at a full meeting of the team but smaller clinics cannot do this. A decision that, when a patient whose condition is not being improved after attending one member of the team for three months be sent automatically to another member of the team, avoids this problem.

(b) Outpatients

Most of the patients attending the pain relief clinic will not differ greatly from outpatients attending any other clinic. However, there will be a greater number of patients who cannot move about easily because of pain, or who are physically handicapped by paraplegia or lower limb amputation. These patients will need special facilities for transportation between outpatient and radiological department, laboratory, other clinics and the toilets; they may indeed require special toilet facilities within easy reach. As a corollary of this there will be the necessity for the ready help of porters and chairs and nurses. There are certain necessities which must be provided; for instance, as examination of the patient is an absolute essential, a suitable examination couch with sufficient space to walk all round it is required. Also, a desk and a chair for the physician to use, sink and water, storage cupboards for instruments and equipment, and a supply of various syringes, needles and solutions conveniently on a trolley. A suitable list is appended (p. 84) but its contents will differ depending on the techniques used in the particular clinic.

(c) Inpatients

There are some requirements that are absolutely necessary for the efficient running of a pain relief centre. The first is that the clinic must have its own beds, that is inpatient beds which belong to and are at the disposal of the physicians of the pain relief centre and cannot be pre-empted by any other physician without prior arrangement with the pain relief physician. Usually a relatively small number of these, say four or five, are sufficient provided other beds can be borrowed when required. Often, when a physician or surgeon calls on the services of the pain relief clinic of his own hospital, his patients are treated in his own beds. For instance, the Centre for Pain Relief at Walton Hospital, Liverpool, has only four beds of its own, but at any one time has up to ten beds occupied by patients under treatment.

A great benefit can be obtained by a pain relief centre when there is a day ward available in the hospital and when beds can be obtained regularly in this. When a day ward is not present, it may be possible to use the beds of ambulant patients in other wards during the day. This can be a very successful method and is used in many hospitals. As mentioned previously, patients who come from a distance will have to stay in the hospital if treatment and investigation is required, but with some types of treatment it is possible for the patient to lodge in a hostel or hotel nearby. Some hospitals have a short stay ward where patients may be admitted for not more than five days and which is not staffed over the weekends. This is an exceedingly useful place for dealing with some patients and conserves staff. Finally, the use of the overnight stay for many patients provides very safe observation when some potentially dangerous procedures are carried out, such as diagnostic coeliac plexus block or diagnostic or semipermanent lumbar sympathetic block. It is particularly desirable to have this facility for the older patient.

(d) Appointment system

An appointment system is absolutely essential for a pain relief centre, but it is not expected that appointments will be rigidly kept, as there is no knowing for sure in advance how difficult it will be to evaluate a particular patient. In arranging patient appointments, the time allowed for each particular patient is to some extent decided by the type of referral accepted by the centre, and also whether the patient has been seen before, i.e. is a new patient or is a follow-up patient. Emergency arrangements will have to be organized so that a patient can be seen urgently (e.g. a severe trigeminal neuralgia), or a special visit of a non-emergency patient can be seen out of ordinary hours (e.g. after travelling a long distance). If the patient to be seen has a straightforward condition needing say injection for rheumatic trigger points or sub-acromial bursitis, or for decision about diagnostic block, then perhaps fifteen minutes only need be allowed. X-ray reports, laboratory reports and previous specialist findings should if possible be obtained before the interview so that time is not wasted waiting for this information. In this way a large number of new patients, say three to four per hour, can be seen. However, if these patients are to be used for teaching purposes, then the time allowed must be increased. When the new patient is not suffering from a simple (probably known) condition, then 45 minutes to 1 hour will be necessary. If the patient has been referred specially, has a long history, and has been treated by many other physicians and centres, then more time than this will be necessary. Follow-ups take fifteen minutes and these average times will allow a simple block to be carried out as well. An approximation is that about one in three visits will require a block of simple type, which can be carried out in the outpatients' department – if the facilities are to hand.

As previously mentioned, some patients turn up at the wrong time, or on the wrong day, or arrive unexpectedly late through no fault of their own. They may have an acute exacerbation of their pain and come to the clinic because of their own or a relative's panic. These patients must be dealt with. The first person to see them after the clerk will be the sister and an experienced nurse in this type of situation will sort out most problems but some of these patients will need to be seen by a doctor. In a large clinic a designated doctor not carrying on the outpatient work that day will be available – 'first on call' for this purpose. In a small clinic a previous arrangement must be made with say the casualty department to see them. Failing any standard arrangement, the patient can either wait to the end of the outpatient clinic or be admitted.

Distinction has to be made between those patients who live within reasonable distance of the clinic and those who come from afar. Patients from a distance will have elastic appointment times, bearing in mind that there is little point in seeing them when hospital facilities such as radiological and laboratory examinations, nerve conduction times are not available and the investigatory departments have closed down for the day. Otherwise the patient will have to return the following day to have these done. All pain relief clinics have to deal with patients who have intermittent pain and who, when they arrive at the clinic, have no pain on that particular day. These patients are usually examined and investigated if their present condition warrants it and then arrangements made for the patient when in pain to phone in to the secretary of the pain relief department who will arrange for him to be seen by a member of the team. If this arrangement is to work, both the patient, secretary and members of the pain team must know what is expected of them. The patient must be warned that on any particular occasion it may not be possible for them to be seen at such short notice, but if they keep on phoning in, sooner or later somebody will be free to see them while the pain is active.

(C) Additional facilities

(a) Outpatient
Naturally, there will be clerical staff available in the larger pain relief clinics for basic organizational purposes such as records, letters to referring physicians, interdepartmental communication, finance, research, trainee rosters, registrar duty roles and other routine work. It will be a function of the head of department or chairman to organize this and the

responsibility of all the team members to make such suggestions as are necessary. The propaganda possibilities of the outpatient department should not be forgotten either for teaching patients or trainee medical and nursing staff. Thus the outpatients' rooms themselves can have various charts on their walls, either of an informative nature for the patient, for instance on how to lift weights, or for the benefit of the physicians examining and treating the patients, and particularly for the benefit of trainees. In a nearby area, a small collection of reference books is often useful.

(b) Unit meetings

Regular meetings of the team members will be made to smooth out any difficulties or problems; these should take place at bimonthly intervals. These meetings will be in addition to a grand round once every week, or, in smaller clinics, once every two to four weeks. During winter months, weekly or two weekly meetings should be held for the whole unit, on specific pain problems. Once per year there should be a unit meeting of the whole department, or at least of its permanent staff. It will include, medical, nursing, ancillary and clerical staff. In addition the consultant pain team should meet from time to time to review progress and decide future policy.

(c) Bed occupancy

The length of stay of patients for the various procedures can be given approximately. For example, a fairly fit patient having a percutaneous cervical cordotomy should be in hospital a minimum of four days, postoperatively. Inpatient time pre-operatively will have to be added on to this, depending on the investigations that are required. The patient for pituitary injection of alcohol should stay in hospital for a minimum of five days post-operatively for a single injection, but, as three injections are usual, a total of three weeks may be necessary. After semi-permanent chemical coeliac plexus block a minimum of two days post-operatively is needed or until any hypotension is controlled. The lumbar sympathetic block patient should stay in overnight, while after intrathecal phenol block hospitalization for a day or two is usually adequate unless complications arise. A patient who is having dorsal column stimulator implant evaluation will take up to two weeks. It should be realized that these measures are only average estimates; they will vary in different pain relief centres and should therefore not be taken as fixed times.

(d) Back-up facilities

In a simple clinic back-up facilities are minimal but a few problems can be envisaged, e.g. who will provide emergency cover during ordinary working hours, at night, during holidays? Who writes up the case history and makes the pre-operative examination when the patient comes to the day ward, or, more rarely, the hospital inpatient ward if there is a more complicated procedure or some special investigation required? In the intermediate sized clinic the problem is easier to solve because there is more than one pain-relief clinician, and in the multidisciplinary clinic there are plentiful medical personnel at all levels. What is more important there will be nurse and ancillary help of various expertise. Nevertheless, duties of resident medical staff must be properly defined and patients provided with effective and expert medical cover at all times.

MANAGEMENT OF A PAIN RELIEF CENTRE

(A) Techniques

One of the tendencies in a pain relief centre is to ignore other methods of treatment. For instance, a patient who has pain from a secondary cancer in bone may best be treated by a palliative dose of radiation. Similarly, it must not be forgotten that chemotherapy, surgery or drug therapy, may provide satisfactory pain relief. It is necessary, therefore, for close ties to be built between these other specialties and the pain relief centre and that specialists from these disciplines should be consulted when required. Ideally there should be an attachment of one each of these specialists to the pain relief centre as apart from pain relief, continuing treatment of the patient by them is necessary. As was mentioned on p. 65 new techniques for pain relief are constantly being devised and these and new equipment need evaluating. A clear and careful idea of when, where, how and by whom such techniques and equipment are to be tested must be known. Only if there is a forum amongst the team members for considering this can the pain relief clinic be managed in the best possible way and offer the best in pain relief. It may well be that one pain relief clinic cannot evaluate all things and so arrangements can be made with other equivalent clinics to share this burden.

(B) Growth of the clinic

The best method of building up a pain relief clinic in Europe is to start by treating cancer pain. This is by far the easiest type of chronic pain to treat, is very satisfying clinically, and most appreciated by other doctors, and not least by the patients and their relatives. Once some good results have been obtained, patients with other types of chronic pain will appear at the clinic. This suggestion does not necessarily hold good for other countries such as the United States of America. It is generally accepted amongst pain relief clinicians that there is far more pain relief work available than there are physicians willing to, or capable of, dealing with it.

A recent publication[25] suggests that after the centre has evaluated the pain problem and worked out the course of treatment for the patient, the treatment itself could be carried out in the community.

There is an early incentive in pain clinics to use auxilliary help where possible. For certain types of work, nurses can and should be specially trained. For instance, in units using transcutaneous electrical nerve stimulation[12,13], (TNS) special training of one or more of the nurses in the correct placing of skin electrodes should be arranged. In the same fashion, when patients are having acupuncture[23] specially trained nurses are useful and helpful. This special training is beyond that which normally takes place when a nurse works with a particular physician or operator and gets used to his or her methods.

The importance of an adequate period of follow-up supervision cannot be overstressed especially in cases with marked 'psychosomatic overlay'. Painter *et al.*[26] report a 25% regression rate following pain clinic treatment.

Auxillary help should be allowed for in a pain relief clinic and in particular for physiotherapist, radiologist, EMG technician and specially trained personnel in the use of biofeedback methods. Often, as the patient requiring biofeedback is also under the care of physiotherapists, the physiotherapy department may well take over the application of biofeedback under medical direction.

Such procedures as acupuncture, TNS and biofeedback need special equipment, and this must be present in sufficient quantity so that more than one patient at a time can be treated when there are sufficient examination rooms for this to be carried out.

(C) Medico-legal problems

There is an increasing tendency throughout the world for the members of the various populations to sue their doctors for anything less than a perfect result. This will result in a tendency for pain relief physicians to treat non-malignant pain by drug therapy, TNS, hypnosis, operant conditioning and other non-invasive methods. The multidisciplinary approach to the pain relief clinic, apart from its usefulness, also protects the participating physicians, as it is difficult to argue in a court of law that, say, six doctors were all wrong in deciding the treatment.

TERMINAL CARE

A unit which undoubtedly serves an important need, and provides a most useful service is the terminal care unit where the situation and attitude is very different to that normally found in hospitals. There is a concentration on making the patient as comfortable as possible during the last period of life and improving the quality of that life. Pain is not the only or even the major problem in a terminal care unit[6], but, because it is an over-riding one, the personnel of the pain relief centre are likely to be involved in it. In fact, considering the benefits that are obtained by such a unit itself, and the benefits pain relief centre clinicians can provide to such a centre, a terminal care unit might reasonably be provided in or near each major hospital, with the pain relief clinic ready to provide advice, help and technical manoeuvres in respect of pain relief. The terminal care unit will be organized and its day to day running carried out by its own personnel[7,27].

References

1 Bonica, J. J. (1951). The role of the anaesthesiologist in the management of intractable pain. *Canad. Anaesth. Soc. J.*, **12,** 103
2 Bonica, J. J. (1953). *The Management of Pain.* (Philadelphia: Lea & Febiger)
3 Bonica, J. J. (1974). Organisation and function of a pain clinic. In Bonica, J. J. (ed.). *Advances in Neurology.* Vol. 4. 433–443
4 Bonica, J. J. (1976). Introduction to the First World Congress on Pain. Goals of the I.A.S.P. and the World Congress. In Bonica, J. J. and Albe-Fessard, D. (eds.) *Advances in Pain Research and Therapy.* Vol. 1. pp. XXVII-XXXIX. (New York: Raven Press)
5 Nayman, J. (1979). Measurement and control of post-operative pain. *Ann. R. Coll. Surg. Engl.*, **61,** 419
6 Hinton, J. M. (1963). The physical and mental distress of the dying. *Q. Med. J.*, **32,** 1
7 Twycross, R. G. (1978). Relief of pain. In Saunders, G. M. (ed.). *The Management of Terminal Disease.* p. 66. (London: Edward Arnold)
8 Bonica, J. J. and Butler, S. H. (1978). The management and functions of pain centres. In Swerdlow, M. (ed.). *Relief of Intractable Pain.* 2nd edn. Chapter 3. pp. 44–50 (Amsterdam: Excerpta Medica)
9 Benn, R. T. and Wood, P. H. N. (1975). Pain in the back. An attempt to estimate the size of the problem. *Rheumatol. Rehabil.*, **14,** 121
10 Twycross, R. G. (1979). Effect of cocaine in the Brompton Cocktail. In Bonica, J. J. *et. al.* (eds.). *Advances in Pain Research and Therapy* Vol. 3 pp. 927–932. (New York: Raven Press)
11 Ventafridda, V., Figluizzi, M. Tamburini, M., Gori, E., Parolaro, D. and Sala, M. (1979). Clinical observations on analgesia elicited by intrathecal morphine in cancer patients. In Bonica, J. J. *et al.* (eds.). *Advances in Pain Research and Therapy.* Vol. 3. pp. 559–565. (New York: Raven Press)

12 Long, D. M., Campbell, J. N. and Gunduz Gucer (1979). Transcutaneous electrical stimulation for relief of chronic pain. In Bonica, J. J. *et al.* (eds.). *Advances in Pain Research and Therapy.* Vol. 3. pp. 593–599 (New York: Raven Press)

13 Anderson, S. A. (1979). Pain Control by Sensory Stimulation. In Bonica, J. J. *et al.* (eds.) *Advances in Pain Research and Therapy.* Vol. 3. pp. 569–585. (New York: Raven Press)

14 Orne, M. T. (1976). Mechanisms of hypnotic pain control. In Bonica, J. J. and Albe-Fessard, D. (eds.) *Advances in Pain Research and Therapy.* Vol. 1. pp. 717–726. (New York: Raven Press)

15 Rose, S. S. and Swerdlow, M. (1980). Pain due to peripheral vascular disease. In Lipton S. (ed.) *Persistent Pain.* Vol. 2. pp. 283–323 (New York and London: Academic Press)

16 Lipton, S. (1979). (ed.) *The Control of Chronic Pain.* Chap. 6. pp. 40–43. (London: Edward Arnold)

17 Swerdlow, M. (1972). The pain clinic. *Br. J. Clin. Pract.,* **26,** 403

18 Swerdlow, M. (1978). The value of clinics for the relief of chronic pain. *J. Med. Ethics,* **4,** 117

19 Mushin. W. W., Swerdlow, M., Lipton S. and Mehta, M. D. (1977). The pain centre. *Practitioner,* **218,** 439

20 Ganz, E. and Mullan, S. (1977). Percutaneous cordotomy. In Lipton, S. (ed.) *Persistent Pain.* Vol. 1, Chap. 2, pp. 22–33. (New York and London: Academic Press)

21 Bond, M. R. (1979). Pain. Its nature, analysis and treatment. Chap. 12. *Pain and Mental Illness.* (Edinburgh: Churchill Livingstone)

22 Mehta, M. and Sluijter, M. E. (1979). The treatment of chronic back pain. A preliminary survey of the effect of radiofrequency denervation of the posterior vertebral joints. *Anaesthesia,* **34,** 8, 768

23 Sjolund, B., Terenius, L. and Erikson, M. (1977). Increased cerebrospinal fluid levels of endorphine after electroacupuncture. *Acta Physiol. Scand.,* **100,** 382

24 Swerdlow, M. (1979). Personal Communication

25 Rockwell, F. P., Rosenblatt, R. and Corkill, G. (1979). Pain clinic model for community practice. *West. J. Med.,* **131,** 166

26 Painter, J. R., Seres, J. L. and Newman, R. I. (1980). Assessing benefits of the pain center; why some patients regress. *Pain,* **8,** 101

27 Twycross, R. G. (1979). Overview of analgesia. In Bonica, J. J. and Ventafridda, V. (eds) *Advances in Pain Research and Therapy.* Vol. 2. pp. 617–633. (New York: Raven Press)

APPENDIX I

Operating Theatre

Lesion generator suitable for:

Percutaneous cordotomy

Trigeminal RFC

Facetectomy

Nerve stimulator

Pituitary injection needle

Pencil torch

Image intensifier
Radio-translucent operating table (with cordotomy headrest)
Lead aprons
Electric skin thermometer

Outpatients
    Separate nerve stimulator
    TNS stimulator
    Acupuncture stimulator
    Acupuncture point detector

Needles and solutions

(I) Needles: Acupuncture ½″, 1″, 2″, ear needles
                  Hypodermic 25 × ½″
                                 23 × 1″
                                 21 × 1½″, 2″, 2½″
                  Paravertebral 20 × 6″, 8″
                  Spinal   18, 20, 22 gauge
                  Tuohy   16, 18 gauge
                  Stimulating (insulated) 2″, 3″, 4″, 6″

(II) Solutions: *Sterilizing fluids*
                    Skin
                    Instruments
                    Local anaesthetic solutions:
                        Lignocaine, ½%, 1%, 2%, plain and with adrenaline
                              1 in 200 000
                        Bupivacaine, 0.25%, 0.5%, plain and with adrenaline
                              1 in 200 000
                    Neurolytic solutions:-
                      Phenol in Myodil, 1 in 15, 1 in 20
                      Phenol in glycerine, 1 in 15, 1 in 20
                      Phenol solution, 2%, 6%
                      Absolute alcohol
                    Chlorocresol, 1 in 50 in glycerine
                                     1 in 40 in glycerine

4

Current views of the pharmacological management of pain

N. E. Williams

INTRODUCTION

Neuro-pharmacological studies are gradually revealing the complexity of the biochemical mechanisms involved in pain. Many known substances may be implicated as 'excitors' of pain production at peripheral sites, and varying levels of a number of known or putative transmitters within the central nervous system appear to influence the transmission and perception of pain. Paradoxical situations, too, can occur: if 5-hydroxytryptamine (serotonin; 5-HT) is applied to a blistered area, intense pain will result, and this substance is also implicated in 'triggering' off a migraine attack. Conversely, elevated levels of 5-hydroxytryptamine within the CNS appear to be most beneficial in modifying both the transmission and the subjective response to pain.

It is therefore not surprising that the pharmacological approach to pain has evolved far beyond the use of drugs which are derivatives or analogues of these extracted from the poppy and the willow bark. A wide variety of drugs, some of which would not normally be considered as analgesics, are now proving of considerable value in the treatment of chronic pain.

Many experts in this field genuinely believe that biochemical modification will be the ultimate answer to pain relief, and new drugs continue to be tried with great enthusiasm. However, a word of caution is felt to be necessary. The problem of the measurement of pathological pain remains incompletely resolved; furthermore the placebo response in pain-relieving procedures may be as high as 30%, and the success of a 'new' drug trial may relate to the enthusiasm and kindly interest shown by the medical attendants to a previously 'neglected' patient with a long-standing pain problem. Nevertheless, carefully controlled clinical trials must be considered the most useful methods by which further progress in the pharmacological management of intractable pain can be attained.

The following discussion includes both long established drugs and those which must still be considered as in an experimental stage in the field of pain relief and possible mechanisms of action are indicated where feasible. A practical clinical range of dosage is given for the various drugs. It is, however, important to bear in mind that the individual dose requirements in patients with chronic pain are very variable, but nevertheless the dose must be tailored to the individual patient.

(1) ANALGESICS

Analgesics are broadly divided into two main groups:
    (A) Narcotic analgesics
    (B) Non-steroidal anti-inflammatory (NSAI) drugs.
    These drugs may relieve many types of pain, and under a wide variety of circumstances, i.e. they are 'non-specific' analgesics.

(A) Narcotic analgesics

The use of the descriptive term 'potent' has often led to considerable confusion in the classification of this group of drugs. In the strict pharmacological sense, potency equates with receptor affinity; thus a knowledge of the equi-analgesic doses of narcotic drugs would suggest that dihydrocodeine is approximately twice as potent as pethidine. From a clinical point of view the 'potency' of these agents has sometimes been related to their liability to produce drug dependence and/or drug abuse. On this basis the potencies of pethidine and dihydrocodeine would be reversed. In this context it is felt therefore that the expressions 'strong' or 'weak' narcotics can be more suitably applied.

Mode of action
Our knowledge of the mode of action of narcotic analgesic drugs has been greatly enhanced by the use of autoradiographic studies. Using a radio-labelled narcotic drug, regional localization of opiate uptake has been demonstrated:—

(1) At a dense band in the spinal cord corresponding to the substantia gelatinosa.
(2) At the brainstem level, in solitary nuclei which receive afferent vagal fibres, and in the area postrema which contains the chemo-receptor trigger zone.

(3) In the cortex, especially in the medial thalamic nuclei which mediate poorly localized and emotionally influenced 'deep' pain; in the periaqueductal grey matter; most abundantly in the amygdaloid nuclei, which may reflect the capacity of narcotic agents to alter the subjective reaction to pain.

The concept of a single type of opiate receptor is confounded by the incompleteness of cross-tolerance between individual narcotics and furthermore by the development of drugs with a mixed agonist/antagonist profile. One theory is that the receptor may change shape (and thus vary its affinity) in relation to extracellular Na^+ concentrations. An alternative hypothesis concerns a multi-receptor system of which the main types are mu (μ) thought to be responsible for euphoria and supraspinal analgesic activity, kappa ($\varkappa$) which relate to spinal analgesia and sedation, and sigma (σ) receptors which account for the dysphoric and hallucinatory effects. A fourth receptor, delta (δ), is sometimes implicated to describe peripheral gut (and possibly central) receptors with high affinity for endogenous peptides. Most morphine-like drugs are thought to exert their agonist activity chiefly at μ receptors; mixed agonist/antagonists are considered to exert their analgesic action via $\varkappa$ receptors, and their main undesirable side effects via σ receptors, whilst producing 'competitive' antagonism at μ receptors. Buprenorphine and profadol, however, may be considered as partial agonists; they appear to have great affinity (and therefore 'high potency') at the μ receptor, but a low intrinsic activity; theoretically, this should result in a relatively long duration of action and a high margin of safety. Finally, the usefulness of naloxone and naltrexone (which are pure antagonists) is now being explored in the field of intractable pain.

Clinical aspects

(1) 'STRONG' NARCOTIC AGONISTS INCLUDE:

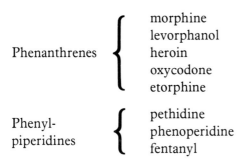

Phenanthrenes	{	morphine levorphanol heroin oxycodone etorphine
Phenyl- piperidines	{	pethidine phenoperidine fentanyl

Methadone and its congeners $\left\{\begin{array}{l}\text{methadone}\\\text{dipipanone}\\\text{dextomoramide}\end{array}\right.$

Benzmorphans   phenazocine

Most pain-relief doctors consider that this group of drugs should be reserved for the treatment of chronic pain associated with recurrent malignancy, when simpler analgesics have become ineffective. Abolition of such pain by alternative methods (e.g. neurolytic blockade, percutaneous cordotomy) often allows rapid withdrawal of high doses of narcotic analgesics with minimum side-effects, suggesting that drug dependency is not a problem. Nevertheless, the continuous use of these drugs in chronic pain conditions where life expectancy is normal is to be deplored.

Morphine

The molecular structure of morphine is represented in its conventional form (Figure 1). A steric arrangement will demonstrate the chair-shaped structure of the methylene bridge (Figure 2).

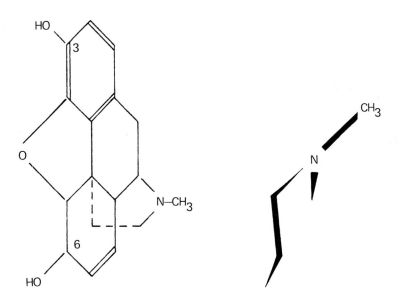

Figure 1   **Figure 2**

This part of the molecule is common to the agonists which appear to be chemically dissimilar and may be the site of attachment to the receptor.

Morphine is considered as having a low oral/parenteral therapeutic ratio. This is presumably due to an extensive clearance of the drug from the portal venous circulation by the liver ('first pass' effect), producing the glucuronide metabolite by conjugation at the 3-OH group. Nevertheless, some workers claim that good pain relief can often be achieved with low doses (e.g. 2.5–5 mg) of oral morphine; furthermore significant blood levels may be attained when slow-release preparations of the drug are used. Presumably, entero-hepatic circulation accounts for the increased availability of morphine.

Heroin owes its superior efficacy to (i) an acetyl group at the 3-carbon position which protects it from the liver microsomal enzymes, (ii) increased lipoid solubility which facilitates transfer across the blood–brain barrier and may account for the high incidence of euphoria. However, this latter side-effect may result from the cocaine which is conventionally used in Brompton type mixtures containing heroin. A world shortage of cocaine, combined with reports that this alkaloid may produce an undue degree of excitation, is now greatly limiting its use in this context. Thus the true role of heroin in the control of pain associated with malignancy may come to be more accurately evaluated. At present, it has connotations of finality–the drug to be used when all others have failed.

Levorphanol remains a popular drug. It is structurally related to morphine, but is 10–15 times as potent by the oral route, and clinical reports suggest that nausea and vomiting are uncommon side-effects. It is available as 1.5 mg tablets.

Oxycodone is slightly less potent than morphine, but has a similar abuse liability. It is well absorbed from the gastrointestinal tract, and the pectinate compound (marketed in the UK as Proladone suppositories which contain the equivalent of 30 mg oxycodone) is probably the drug of choice for rectal administration.

Etorphine is approximately 200 times more potent than morphine when used in man and has undergone limited clinical trials in cancer patients. Despite claims of a decreased incidence of undesirable side-effects as compared with morphine, it has not become generally available.

Phenazocine the benzmorphan derivative, is well absorbed orally, and more recently has been recommended for sub-lingual administration; 5 mg tablets are used.

Pethidine and its related compounds are of little value in the present context. Limited oral absorption and extensive biotransformation markedly reduce their efficiency.

Methadone and related compounds exhibit superior oral efficiency. Analgesia occurs within 20–30 minutes following the ingestion of methadone, and it has an extended duration of action, presumably because it is bound to tissue protein; it is also less constipating than morphine. Five mg tablets, or a syrup containing 2 mg methadone in 5 ml, may be utilized. However, the drug should be used with caution in the elderly or extremely debilitated patient, as cumulation is liable to occur.

Dextromoramide and *dipipanone*, both have a shorter duration of action than methadone. Dipipanone is usually marketed with the antiemetic cyclizine (Diconal – each tablet containing 10 mg dipipanone and 30 mg cyclizine) and is of proven value. Dextromoramide is claimed by the manufacturers to produce less constipation than other narcotic drugs; available preparations of this drug are 5 mg and 10 mg tablets and a suppository containing 10 mg.

Narcotic drugs in the management of cancer pain
Ideally, the pharmacological management of a patient with cancer pain should consist of oral administration of:

(1) The narcotic analgesic which produces the minimum of undesirable side effects.
(2) The minimal dose of this drug necessary to ensure adequate pain relief.
(3) The drug given at sufficiently frequent intervals to prevent the return of 'severe' pain.

Individual variations in response to the drugs in this group may be quite marked, especially in relation to such undesirable side-effects as dysphoria, constipation, nausea and vomiting. 'Ringing the changes' may lead one to the most suitable drug to use. Tolerance and dependence are likely to ensue when any of these drugs is used for 2–3 weeks. Tolerance is initially counteracted by increasing the dosage and frequency of the analgesic administration, but changing to another drug may be of value in re-establishing pain control and has the additional advantage of delaying habituation.

Route of administration – In general, narcotics will be administered orally as long as this is feasible. The regular use of the intramuscular route should be avoided if at all possible; the cancer patient may become demoralized due to further reliance upon medical attendants and abcesses may develop at the site of intramuscular injection in cachectic individuals. In addition, the alteration in shape of the time–effect curve which occurs with parenteral administration means that more frequent dosage is necessary. However, a long acting preparation Duromorph, a micro-crystalline suspension of morphine 64 mg/ml may be used when indicated to minimize some of these disadvantages.

When swallowing is difficult, more *palatable preparations* (syrups) will be indicated. Alternatively, the *sub-lingual* route may be used; this avoids the 'first-pass' effect, and allows a more rapid and enhanced drug action. It may be especially suitable just prior to a period of increased activity (e.g. travelling, bathing, physiotherapy).

Rectal absorption of narcotics may be slow but nevertheless, when used last thing at night (e.g. to supplement oral therapy) they may help to delay early re-awakening due to pain.

The discovery of the existence of opiate receptors in the substantia gelatinosa of the spinal cord has led to a developing interest in the *subarachnoid and epidural* administration of narcotic analgesics. Selective uptake of these drugs by spinal cord receptors at the appropriate dermatomal levels should, theoretically, have immense practical advantages, viz:

(1) Because of 'localization' of the drug, only small doses need to be used.
(2) Avoidance of systemic enzymatic activity should ensure a prolonged duration of action of the drug.
(3) Undesirable side-effects should be minimal due to lack of supra-spinal activity.
(4) Motor weakness, as seen with the similar usage of local anaesthetics and neurolytic agents, should not occur.

In practice the clinical value of this technique is not yet clear. Published reports have shown, on intrathecal injection, of narcotic agents with a high lipoid solubility (e.g. pethidine and its congeners) may be more completely taken up by nervous tissue than morphine. There are obvious practical drawbacks to the repeated use of the subarachnoid route.

If the extradural route is chosen, direct diffusion of the drug across the dura into the cerebrospinal fluid (CSF) is assumed to occur. Personal experience suggests that this method may be of value in the terminal patient with otherwise unmanageable pain. The study was carried out using morphine which has low lipid solubility; at this site uptake of lipoid-soluble drugs by extradural fat may be significant. Doses of 1–2 mg diluted with up to 10 ml of isotonic saline, were injected via an indwelling epidural catheter at 8–10 hourly intervals. Adequate pain relief was attained in three patients for 7–10 days, when tolerance to the drug became evident. Itching over the site of the injection frequently occurs when the spinal route is used; early and 'delayed onset' respiratory depression have been described and catatonic seizure has been reported when larger doses of the narcotic have been employed in an attempt to combat tolerance.

(2) 'WEAK' NARCOTIC AGONISTS INCLUDE:

> Codeine
> Dihydrocodeine
> Dextropropoxyphene
> Ethoheptazine

Codeine is structurally very similar to morphine, but owes its superior oral efficacy to the 'protection' by a methyl group at the 3-carbon atom position. The drug has a low abuse potential, and large doses tend to produce excitation rather than depression; it also has a marked constipating effect. Small doses (5–10 mg) of the drug are commonly incorporated, along with NSAIs, into analgesic compounds used in the treatment of pain of moderate intensity.

The use of *dihydrocodeine* in the treatment of chronic pain is well-established, and in many cases it may be considered as the drug of choice. It can be most effective in a wide variety of painful conditions and drug dependence and abuse are unlikely; in addition, like other narcotic drugs and unlike NSAIs, toxic effects of a 'cellular' nature are not seen with long-term use. Thirty mg tablets may be prescribed on a 4–6 hourly basis. Constipation may be a troublesome side-effect, and dizziness, which is presumably due to increased vestibular sensitivity, can be a problem in the ambulant patient.

Dextropropoxyphene is chemically related to methadone and has been used alone or in compound preparations; a popular formulation in the UK in recent years has been *Distalgesic,* each tablet containing 325 mg paracetamol and 32.5 mg dextropropoxyphene. It has now become evident that the drug is not without risk; some degree of dependence can occur, and a number of incidents of drug abuse, particularly in combination with alcohol, have been reported. In addition, over-dosage or drug interaction may lead to the rapid development of profound respiratory depression which will precede the manifestations of paracetamol hepatoxicity. Nevertheless, a number of patients, particularly with cancer pain or pain due to post-herpetic neuralgia, appear to gain considerable benefit from the use of this compound. If special precautions are taken with respect to maximum daily dosage and possible interaction with other respiratory depressant drugs, it can be of some value. Clinical trials with *Ethoheptazine* have indicated that it fares little better than placebo in relieving pain; however, it is commonly incorporated into compounds containing aspirin or paracetamol, and may have a 'supra-additive' effect.

(3)   MIXED AGONIST/ANTAGONISTS:

Pentazocine (25–50 mg tablets) was the first drug in this group to be promoted for clinical use as an analgesic. It may induce withdrawal symptoms in patients who have been taking opiates on a regular basis and it would therefore seem unwise to use a regime which involves a combination of these drugs. It is not very effective in relieving severe pain. As with other drugs in this group, psychomimetic effects, such as bizarre dreams and hallucinations, may be a problem; nausea and vomiting are common, and myopathy has been reported following prolonged use. *Butorphanol* appears to produce less undesirable side effects than pentazocine when used in the management of post-operative pain; unfortunately it is only available in the UK as a parental preparation at present. *Nalbuphine* has been evaluated as an analgesic in cancer patients. It appears to be approximately four times as potent as pentazocine, and has a slower onset of action though a more prolonged effect when used by the parenteral route. The proposal that drugs of this group may have a special affinity for spinal (x) receptors suggests that they may be particularly indicated when the intrathecal or extradural route of administration is contemplated.

(4)   PARTIAL AGONISTS

Buprenorphine is more appropriately considered under this heading. Its avidity for, but low intrinsic activity at, the μ receptors suggests a relatively long duration of action, a wide margin of safety, and avoidance of psychomimetic effects. Clinical observation suggests that cumulation and respiratory depression may occur when repeated doses of the drug are given by parenteral routes, and this effect is not easily reversed by naloxone. However, a trial of sub-lingual buprenorphine in cancer pain, using doses of 0.15–0.8 mg suggests that it may be a useful addition to the range of drugs available. Drowsiness is commonly seen, but it lessens with continued usage of the drug, and constipation does not occur.

(5)   'PURE' NARCOTIC ANTAGONISTS:

Naloxone (and naltrexone) were developed for use in clinical practice in the treatment of narcotic poisoning and for the prevention of dependence on such drugs; they were originally considered to be devoid of any action *per se* on nociception. However, animal experiments have shown that low doses of naloxone can decrease the latencies to reflex responses of mice or rats which were subjected to the hot-plate test and which had not previously been exposed to opiate drugs. It has been proposed that this effect is due to antagonism of the endogenous peptide system, or is part of a generalized 'excitatory' process. Both these concepts are possibilities as naloxone:

(a) Appears to reverse analgesia produced by classical Chinese acupuncture or placebo medication.
(b) Has been used successfully in the treatment of poisoning by other CNS depressants such as alcohol.

Conversely, large doses of naloxone (4–8 mg) may have beneficial effects in chronic pain states. Some patients with central pain associated with ischaemic lesions of the brainstem ('thalamic syndrome') have reported marked diminution or disappearance of an otherwise refractory pain when this drug has been used intravenously. In this context, naloxone must be used with some caution as cardiac arrhythmias and psychomimetic effects may occur.

(B) Non-steroidal anti-inflammatory drugs (NSAIs)

Mode of action
These drugs, which are also termed the antipyretic analgesics, are considered to exert their main pain-relieving action at peripheral sites. Classically, they have been shown to modify nociceptive responses induced by the polypeptide *bradykinin*. Activation of the kinin-forming system can be induced by tissue injury. The hyperaemia, oedema and pain of an inflammatory response can all be mediated by bradykinin, and the peptide can be identified in inflammatory exudates and synovial fluid from arthritic joints. This class of drugs is known for its efficiency in the relief of mild to moderate pain of a superficial, somatic origin, and where there is often evidence of tissue injury (e.g. arthritides, musculo-skeletal injuries, toothache); their analgesic action could therefore rightly be assumed to be an extension of the anti-inflammatory effect.

Recently interest has centred upon the role of these drugs in inhibiting the enzymatic synthesis of prostaglandins (PGs) from long-chain fatty acids. In man, the sub-dermal infusion of PGE_1 and PGE_2 will produce oedema and a lowered pain threshold to artificial stimuli, although spontaneous pain will not occur. However, if bradykinin (or histamine) is infused as well, intense pain will result. Experimental studies in dogs have suggested that bradykinin may cause release of prostaglandins from the spleen. The accumulated evidence indicates that prostaglandins of the E series, which are produced at the site of injury, may sensitize the peripheral nerves to other mediators such as bradykinin.

Certain malignant tumours, particularly of the breast (but also of lung, kidney and prostate) can produce substantial amounts of PG-like material. It has been shown that some prostaglandins are potent bone-resorbing agents. It is therefore feasible that such tumour cells, on entering bone, may initiate bone resorption. The resultant increase in extracellular calcium and phosphate ions locally may induce pain (as is assumed to occur in Paget's disease); at the same time the formation of metastases may be facilitated. It would therefore seem logical to use NSAIs in the treatment of bone pain associated with disseminated malignancy, and indeed they are often highly effective. It is not yet clear whether they have any effect on the progress of the underlying disease.

There is little doubt that there is a central component in the analgesic action of these drugs. Experimentally, a pain response evoked in spinal rats requires greater amounts of aspirin for suppression than in an intact animal. Prostaglandins are found in the central nervous system and are putative transmitters whose production is thought to be influenced by the anterior pituitary hormone, prolactin. In addition, pyrogens increase the synthesis of PGEs in the hypothalamus, which is the site of the antipyretic action of these drugs.

Individual drugs
Aspirin. In addition to the aforementioned mechanisms, aspirin may also exert its analgesic activity via:

(a) A 'cellular' effect (uncoupling of oxidative phosphorylation).
(b) A plasma protein effect, by displacing and liberating free tryptophan from binding sites.
(c) A 'haematological' effect – by an anti-thromboxane action and possibly hypoprothrombinaemia it will reduce platelet 'stickiness' and the resultant production of 5-hydroxytryptamine, itself a known inciter of migraine and allied neuralgias.

Aspirin is an excellent drug; its use has perhaps been clouded by an undue concern with its gastrointestinal side-effects, and paradoxically, by its ready availability. Like all other members of this group, it is well absorbed orally, and it is useful in a wide variety of chronic pain syndromes, particularly those involving musculo-skeletal disorders, and as a 'background' drug in the treatment of trigeminal neuralgia and other facial pains. Preparations of aspirin containing 300–500 mg aspirin in each tablet are available; many of these are incorporated into compounds which also contain a weak narcotic analgesic; the resultant 'supra-additive' effect may be advantageous. Nevertheless, problems may occur. Hypersensitivity reactions may produce severe gastric bleeding, and a peptic ulcer may be exacerbated. Significant drug interactions, particularly with warfarin anticoagulants and oral antidiabetic agents must be borne in mind. Long-term therapy may lead to the development of analgesic nephropathy.

Various formulations of aspirin are available which may lessen the risks of gastric irritation, either by improving the solubility of the drug and facilitating its distribution across the gastric mucosa, or by increasing the rate of passage into, and subsequent absorption from, the upper intestine. Tablets incorporating alkaline salts of calcium or sodium are available, as well as a polymeric condensation product of aluminium oxide and aspirin – *aloxiprin.*

Diflunisal is a derivative of aspirin which has a longer duration of action than the parent drug. It has little advantage over aspirin, although it may have some value in the management of a patient who is disturbed at night by arthritic pain, or in the prevention of early morning stiffness. The recommended dosage is 250–500 mg twice daily.

Paracetamol which is conventionally included in this group because of its marked antipyretic effect, appears to be devoid of anti-inflammatory activity, although it is said to inhibit the synthesis of certain prostaglandins. However, its therapeutic indications appear to be similar to those for aspirin and as it does not produce gastrointestinal problems, it may be a logical alternative; furthermore the two drugs are frequently incorporated into the same compound, (the range varies from 200 to 500 mg paracetamol in each tablet). *Benorylate* is an ester of aspirin and paracetamol and is thought to be absorbed as such, the free drugs then being released by plasma enzymes. The problem of gastric irritation and bleeding produced by the action of free acetylsalicyclic acid appears to be considerably reduced, but not, as might be expected, completely eliminated.

Paracetamol hepatotoxicity is becoming an increasing problem. Although this is a manifestation of acute overdosage, it has been reported as following the ingestion of as little as 5 g of the drug. Enzyme-inducing drugs, by increasing the production of the toxic axyl metabolites, will further lower the margin of safety. With these provisos, it can be considered a relatively safe and useful drug; however, although there is no evidence that it has any narcotic activity, dependence has occasionally been reported.

Phenylbutazone and indomethacin exhibit powerful anti-inflammatory activity. However, they are the most toxic members of this group, and are less efficient analgesics than salicylates for pain of non-inflammatory origin. Their long-term use should be limited to the management of rheumatoid arthritis, ankylosing spondylitis and allied conditions. A short course of treatment appears to be valuable in the treatment of bone pain associated with malignancy, and indomethacin, through PG synthetase inhibition, has been shown to be effective in the treatment of post-radiation diarrhoea.

Naproxen appears to have a lower incidence of gastrointestinal side effects that some of the older anti-inflammatory drugs. The recommended dose is 250 mg b.d. It has a high affinity for plasma protein and may potentiate the action of anticoagulants, hydantoins and certain sulphonamides. Likewise, *mefenamic acid*, although apparently less harmful to the gut may cause some dyspepsia, drowsiness and diarrhoea, and skin rashes, leukopenia and haemolytic anaemia have been reported. The usual dose is 250–500 mg. t.d.s.

Ibuprofen, and the related compounds *Ketoprofen* and *Flurbiprofen* may be suitable alternatives to aspirin, particularly when drug interactions are a problem. However, as with all these drugs except paracetamol, gastro-intestinal side-effects may still occur.

Nefopam cannot be included in either the narcotic or the NSAI groups. This drug is chemically related to diphenhydramine, and is claimed to be free from narcotic side effects such as habituation and respiratory depression. Nefopam possesses anticholinergic activity and blocks reuptake of noradrenaline. It is available in tablet (30 mg) and injection (20 mg/ml) form, and has been used with some success in the management of musculo-skeletal and cancer pains. The peripheral atropine-like effects may limit its usefulness.

(2) PSYCHOTROPIC DRUGS

(A) Major tranquillizers
Phenothiazines. Chlorpromazine was first synthesized in 1952. It potentiates the activity of a number of analgesics and CNS depressants and is remarkably effective in the relief of agitation and anxiety in schizophrenia. A number of other substituted phenothiazines have subsequently

been introduced into clinical practice. These have shown varying degrees of selectivity with relation to antipsychotic, sedative, antiemetic, extrapyramidal and peripheral activity, and some of them have gained a valuable role as adjuncts in chronic pain therapy.

Some phenothiazines are considered to have an analgesic action per se although with the exception of *methotrimeprazine* (levomepromazine) this has not been proved. These drugs have marked sedative and peripheral effects; the analgesic effect may be part of a generalized 'deafferentation' involving the reticular activating system. Nevertheless it is suggested that methotrimeprazine can be as effective as morphine in equi-analgesic doses; furthermore, when therapy is instituted, tolerance to the sedative and hypotensive effects appear within 48 hours, whereas the analgesic effect persists. Further trials may be indicated, as it is well-known that schizophrenic patients on long-term therapy may remain blissfully unaware of the nociceptive impulses arising from a perforated viscus or a fracture of the femoral neck! Drug dependence of the narcotic variety should not occur; however, other problems such as extrapyramidal disorders or cholestatic jaundice may be anticipated with long-term therapy.

Phenothiazine will be of value when pain (in particular 'atypical' facial pain) is considered as a manifestation of a psychotic delusion, and are also most useful for symptomatic treatment in the agitated cancer patient. In smaller doses, they are frequently used in combination with tricyclic antidepressants in the management of post-herpetic neuralgia and other non-malignant intractable pain conditions (see later).

A thioxanthene analogue of chlorpromazine, *chlorprothixine* has been studied in patients with chronic pain. Although in most cases the unpleasant side-effects outweighed the benefit achieved, a few patients obtained continued pain relief for some months following cessation of therapy.

Butyrophenones are neuroleptic drugs which have similar properties to phenothiazines. They exhibit no inherent analgesic activity, but are more potent dopamine antagonists, and thus their antiemetic and potentiating effects are valuable when they are used in conjunction with narcotic analgesics; *haloperidol* is the drug of choice in this context. A closely related drug is *pimozide*, a long-acting neuroleptic with highly selective and potent dopamine-antagonist properties. It is at present undergoing trials for the relief of chronic pain.

Prochlorperazine and *perphenazine* are strong antiemetics, but produce a lesser degree of sedation and peripheral activity. They are commonly used in conjunction with narcotic analgesics (normally in a dose of 5 mg) to reduce the incidence of vomiting. They appear to potentiate the analgesic and respiratory depressant effect of the narcotic drugs: this may be partly explained by their action in blocking receptors in the chemoreceptor trigger zone, thus allowing a greater portion of the narcotic administered to reach other opiate receptors.

(B)   Antidepressants

Tricyclic antidepressants. These drugs have the ability to:

(1)   Increase the availability of noradrenaline and 5-HT as central transmitters by blocking their neuronal re-uptake.
(2)   Block noradrenaline uptake at post-synaptic receptors (which may relate to their sedative effects).
(3)   Produce atropine-like side-effects due to a central reduction of parasympathetic output.

Pain may be the presenting symptom of a depressive illness or, on the other hand, secondary depression of mood due to physical disease tends to reduce tolerance of pain. Furthermore, descending fibres involving serotonergic pathways are thought to be important in raising the pain threshold, presumably by modifying C-fibre input at the substantia gelatinosa. (The 5-HT precursor, *L-tryptophan* has proved useful in re-establishing control of pain in a patient with an implanted cerebral electrode). The use of these drugs in chronic pain conditions is therefore most logical in addition to their mood elevating effect.

Apart from their obvious value in pain associated with endogenous or reactive depression (e.g. cancer, post-traumatic pain) they have also proved useful in conditions, such as facial pain or low-back pain where depression, although suspected, is not obvious. Their greatest benefit has been in the relief of the severe burning dysaesthesia associated with post-herpetic neuralgia.

Choice of drug

Clinically these drugs vary in relation to:

(1)   Speed of onset of action
(2)   Sedative effects
(3)   Atropine-like effects

Amitriptyline takes 10–14 days to act fully, and exhibits sedative and parasympatholytic effects. Nevertheless, it has been the drug most widely used and is often extremely effective. The sedative effect may be useful in

101

re-establishing a normal sleep pattern when sleep is disturbed by pain. However, the atropine-like side effects may be particularly troublesome and irritating, especially as they may present before any significant pain relief occurs. Personal experience suggests that *protriptyline*, which has a shorter latent period, may be slightly superior. *Imipramine* may be particularly valuable when reversal of anergia is required. *Clomipramine*, which is said to have a more selective action on 5-HT uptake, has also been widely recommended.

The analgesic effect is said to improve markedly if the tricyclic drug of choice is used in combination with a phenothiazine. Some potentiation may occur as hydroxylation of the tricyclic may be inhibited. Marked side-effects may be anticipated but the problem may be minimized by:

(1) Careful explanation to the patient
(2) Withdrawing concurrent drug therapy if this is possible
(3) Starting on a low dose initially (preferably in the evening) and gradually building up to the required therapeutic regime
(4) Reducing the tendency to poor patient compliance by using a simple regime. In this instance, a compound preparation, such as *amitriptyline* and *perphenazine* (Triptafen) may be valuable.

Even when all such precautions are taken, however, there will be a significant incidence of untoward effects, which may considerably outweigh any advantage gained. Furthermore, long-term therapy will usually be necessary as stopping the regime may result in a return of the pain syndrome; the likelihood of toxic effects such as cardiac arrhythmias is thus enhanced. For these reasons, many pain clinicians consider that antidepressant drugs should only be prescribed when the pain is associated with overt signs of depression, and that their routine use in pain therapy is not recommended. It is unfortunate that *mianserin*, a tetracyclic antidepressant whose mode of action at the synapses is unclear but which exhibits minimal peripheral side-effects has not proved more valuable in this context.

Monamine oxidase inhibitors have had some value in management of refractory cases of migraine and other neuralgias, but side-effects and interactions with other drugs and foodstuffs tend to preclude the more general use of these drugs for chronic pain.

(3) ANTICONVULSANTS

A number of drugs which were originally introduced into clinical practice for the treatment of epilepsy have found a valuable role in the management of chronic pain.

These include Carbamazepine

          Diphenylhydantoin (phenytoin)

          Clonazepam

          Sodium valproate

Mode of action

Drugs of this group have found most value in the treatment of trigeminal neuralgia. The paroxysmal nature of this pain allows it to be considered as a type of 'focal' epilepsy, and their 'membrane-stabilizing' activity particularly with respect to the spinal trigeminal nucleus may be of prime importance. An alternative view is that tic douloureux is a pain of central origin i.e. a 'localized' form of thalamic pain. If this is the case, any effect of these drugs in modifying neurotransmitter activity within the CNS may play a part in their action. Carbamazepine is chemically related to the tricyclic antidepressants and will increase brain levels of 5-HT, and some elevation of mood can occur with its use. Valproate can produce increased brain levels of the known inhibitory transmitter, gamma-aminobutyric acid.

However, it has now become clear that anticonvulsant drugs may be effective in a wide range of painful conditions in addition to trigeminal neuralgia, which involve the occurrence of 'stabbing' or 'shooting' pains sometimes accompanied by muscular jerks and twitches. These unpleasant symptoms may be a component of the pain of post-herpetic neuralgia, but may also occur with a variety of painful conditions following surgery or trauma. In such conditions, there is frequently evidence of peripheral nerve damage, and it is postulated that anticonvulsants exert their effect by suppressing abnormal hyperexcitability and discharge to other neuron pools, which occurs in the unmyelinated pain conducting fibres.

The chosen anticonvulsant is started at a low dose level and gradually built up until an effective dosage is attained. Monitoring the blood level during the build-up will help to ascertain achievement of an effective level especially with phenytoin and will detect the occasional patient who does

Table 1 Effective blood levels of anticonvulsants

Drug	Effective blood level (μmol/l)	
	Range	*Mean*
Phenytoin	5–35	16.2
Carbamazepine	9–35	20.6
Sodium valproate	250–720	399
Clonazepam	not available	

not in fact take his tablets. Table 1 shows the range of blood levels required for analgesia; it will be seen that they are lower than those employed against epilepsy.

If the first drug tried produces intolerable side-effects or inadequate analgesia, one of the other anticonvulsants should be tried. When satisfactory relief is obtained the anticonvulsant may need to be taken for a considerable length of time, although in some cases medication can be stopped without recurrence of pain.

It is important to remember that abrupt cessation of long-term anticonvulsant therapy may induce epileptiform attacks. Gradual withdrawal of these drugs is therefore considered mandatory.

Carbamazepine is the drug of choice in the treatment of trigeminal neuralgia. It is so highly effective if it is used correctly that it may almost be considered as a diagnostic tool as well as a therapeutic agent. However, if satisfactory results are to be achieved, the drug must be taken on a regular basis and the dosage may need to be increased to gain the required therapeutic effect. Many of the patients who claim little or no benefit from its use are discovered, on close questioning, to be taking it on an occasional basis and during an attack of spasm. Tolerance to the effect of the drug may occur. This may be due to a real increase in the severity of the condition; alternatively, alteration in the pharmacokinetics of the drug may be the cause, as it is known that carbamazepine can stimulate its own metabolism. In both cases, a further increase in the drug dose may be indicated; a wide variation in the daily requirement of this drug (200–1000 mg) may thus occur.

However, like all other drugs with CNS activity, side-effects may be a problem, and drowsiness and ataxia are common, although these may disappear on continued dosage, and gastric upsets may occur. Occasionally more serious effects, such as bone marrow depression and thrombocytopenia, are seen and regular blood counts are indicated for those patients who receive long-term therapy.

Phenytoin is a logical alternative to carbamazepine. However, it is less effective in trigeminal neuralgia; furthermore it has a narrow therapeutic range and obeys zero-order kinetics, so that toxic plasma levels are all too easily attained; lateral nystagmus is an early sign of overdosage. One approach to this problem is to obtain a reliable plasma phenytoin estimation following a subtherapeutic dose of the drug and then predict from a nomogram the required dose increase necessary. Alternatively, salivary concentrations can be measured. Dose requirements will vary from 100–300 mg daily.

Clonazepam is a benzodiazepine which has been developed for its anti-convulsant activity. Like other members of this group, it is of low toxicity, but tends to produce a marked degree of drowsiness. The initial daily dose should not exceed 1 mg.

Valproate has undergone substantial trial in the treatment of trigeminal neuralgia and is of proven value in the treatment of other lancinating pains mentioned previously. It has been used in conjunction with tricyclic anti-depressants in the treatment of postherpetic neuralgia. It appears to be less toxic than carbamazepine and phenytoin, although disturbances of liver function have been reported; the incidence of gastric irritation may be reduced by the use of a syrup preparation or an enteric-coated capsule. A therapeutic regime may involve using 400–1200 mg daily.

(4) MUSCLE RELAXANTS

Patients with painful reflex muscular hypertonicity may gain some help from centrally acting muscle relaxants.

The benzodiazepines, particularly *diazepam*, have proved valuable in the management of muscle contraction headaches, which are steady, non-pulsatile aches occurring in any region of the cranium, often associated with emotional stress and frequently with tenderness in cranial musculature. These drugs exert a minor tranquillizing effect via the limbic system and reticular formation, but also depress polysynaptic reflexes in the spinal cord and maximally at the site of the reticular formation. A dose of 2–5 mg t.d.s. can be recommended in this context. *Orphenadrine* citrate, whose related hydrochloride salt is used in the treatment of Parkinsonism, and *meprobamate* are suitable alternatives. It is marketed as 100 mg slow-release tablets for twice daily use.

Haloperidol may be used in the treatment of painful episodes associated with spasmodic torticollis. In addition to the tranquillizing effect, it may depress noxious reflexes arising in the basal ganglia. Small doses (1–2 mg daily) should be prescribed.

In multiple sclerosis and other demyelinating diseases, as well as following spinal injury, painful spasms may occur due to the generation of 'toxic' reflexes in polysynaptic pathways within the spinal cord. *Baclofen* which is an analogue of gamma-aminobutyric acid, a known inhibitory transmitter within the CNS, will reduce muscle tone, clonus and spasm in such cases without producing undue cortical depression. A small dose is used initially (5 mg t.d.s.) and is gradually increased until the required therapeutic effect is obtained with a maximum of 40–60 mg daily. An alternative choice is *dantrolene* which is thought to bind Ca^{2+} to the sarcoplasmic reticulum of the muscle, and thus inhibit the formation of the contractile actinomyosin complex (the drug is also useful in the treatment of malignant hyper-pyrexia). Again a gradually increasing dose regime ranging from 25 to 400 mg a day is recommended; a number of cases of hepatotoxicity have been reported with long-term use of the drug.

When intractable pain is associated with recurrent spasm of smooth muscle, drugs with a predominantly peripheral site of action should be chosen. Atropine-like drugs which are quaternary ammonium com-pounds, and therefore do not cross the blood—brain barrier easily, such as *hyoscine hydrobromide* or *propantheline* are useful; a ganglion blocking action may contribute to the effect. Alternatively, drugs with a direct action on smooth muscle ('papaverine-like' effect) such as *mebeverine* can be used.

(5) MISCELLANEOUS DRUGS

Drugs used in the treatment of migraine

Current views of the causation of migraine suggest that an initial release of 5-HT triggers off the vasoconstriction and the associated prodromal symptoms; a further release of 5-HT may occur from platelet aggregation in the constricted vessels. The painful phase, correlating with vasodilat-ation of the extracranial vessels, appears to be mediated via an increased production of histamine and plasma kinins whilst concurrently there is a fall in the plasma 5-HT level. There are thus several approaches to rational drug therapy.

In the acute attack, NSAI drugs, particularly those which inhibit platelet stickiness, are obviously valuable. Vasoconstrictor drugs which act by stimulating peripheral x-receptors, such as *ergotamine* 1–2 mg are also useful. These two types of drugs are frequently used in combination; an antihistamine, such as *buclizine* may also be incorporated, and such compounds if taken at an early stage may abort or considerably modify an attack.

For continuous prophylaxis, *methysergide*, a potent 5-HT antagonist has been used although serious side-effects, in particular the development of retroperitoneal fibrosis, are a problem. A dose of 6 mg daily should not be exceeded, and therapy should be discontinued for at least 1 month in every 6 months. *Cyproheptadine* exhibits both anti-5-HT and antihistamine activity, but although it is less toxic than methysergide it appears to be less effective. More promise has been shown by the introduction of *pizotifen*, which antagonizes plasma kinin as well as histamine and 5-HT activity; so far no serious side-effects have been reported with the use of this drug. The antihypertensive drug *clonidine*, used in smaller doses of 50–150 μg per day, may also be valuable, particularly when the attacks appear to be triggered by the ingestion of foodstuffs containing tyramine.

Propranolol is sometimes useful in the prophylactic treatment of migraine and allied conditions including 'cluster headaches'. One explanation of its effectiveness may be blockade of β-receptors on the pineal body. This organ, which is deemed to be outside the blood–brain barrier, contains large stores of 5-HT. A central sedative effect and an effect on local blood flow mediated via β_2-receptor blockade, may also be implicated. It has also been tried in the treatment of phantom limb pains and 'odd' peripheral pains and is worthy of further controlled trials. However, certain side-effects, such as bronchospasm, peripheral vascular insufficiency and a tendency to produce nightmares, will limit its use. A dose range of 40–120 mg daily is recommended.

Drugs used in causalgia

The painful dysaesthesia associated with peripheral nerve injuries and other traumatic dystrophies is frequently alleviated by sympathetic ganglion blockade. Evidence of increased sympathetic activity in the painful area is frequently elicited in such cases; it therefore seems logical that regional sympatholysis via the adrenergic nerve terminals could be helpful, presumably by interfering with a loop feed-back system involving noradrenaline. Perfusion of a limb isolated under tourniquet and using *guanethidine* is frequently performed in this context. Guanethidine appears to displace noradrenaline from its bound complex and then deplete the nerve terminal by preventing further storage of noradrenaline. Significant pain relief frequently occurs; unfortunately, the effect is usually temporary (3–4 days), although it is claimed that more permanent relief can be attained when the procedure is repeated regularly. *Reserpine* has also been used, but appears to be less effective. If it could be ensured that experimental drugs such as *6-hydroxydopamine* did not escape into the systemic circulation, they could be extremely valuable in this context.

Drugs in peripheral vascular disease

Drugs are of little value in the treatment of intermittent claudication. Alpha-receptor blocking drugs may make the condition worse by diverting blood flow from muscle to skin. β_2-receptor stimulators, such as *isoxuprine*, are more likely to produce vasodilatation in blood vessels supplying skeletal muscle, and may be of some benefit. Various derivatives of nicotinic acid that can relax smooth muscle, and *naftidrofuryl* which also has local anaesthetic activity, have also been advocated; they are more efficacious in the relief of painful conditions associated with reduced skin blood flow, such as Raynaud's phenomenon, acrocyanosis and chilblains.

(6) CURRENT DEVELOPMENTS

Calcitonin. The synthetic preparation of this hormone, salmon calcitonin, is most effective in the treatment of Paget's disease, as it suppresses bone resorption and calcium release; concurrently there is marked relief of bone pain. *Mithramycin*, an antibiotic with cytotoxic activity, has also been shown to have a consistent effect in this disease in producing a biochemical improvement and symptomatic relief. It has recently been suggested that calcitonin may also be highly effective in alleviating pain from other bony diseases, such as osteoporosis or skeletal metastases. A localized fall in PO_4 may be responsible for this effect, as drugs which may release PO_4 such as fosfestrol (Honvan) and hydrocortisone sodium phosphate are prone to produce marked peripheral pain following intravenous injection. In this context high doses of salmon calcitonin (400 IU b.d. for 2 days) may prove valuable.

Phenylalanine. Our knowledge of the existence of endogenous opioid peptides has not yet been a great source of pharmacological advancement in the chronic pain field. However, it has been suggested that the amino acid d-phenylalanine may exert pain-relieving activity in animals and man by inhibiting carboxypeptidase-A, an enzyme concerned in the breakdown of encephalins and endorphins. Results with this substance and with related enzyme inhibitors remain unconfirmed, but further studies are indicated.

Bromocriptine. In pain of central origin associated with vascular lesions involving the thalamus, the use of drugs which may replenish dopaminergic activity would appear rational. Such drugs will also act at hypothalamic levels to inhibit prolactin release, which itself increases CNS prostaglandin levels. Preliminary trials have not so far been encouraged, but the dopamine precursor *L-dopa* might be considered a more suitable alternative. It has been demonstrated that patients with Parkinsonism established on L-dopa therapy exhibit increased pain thresholds and pain tolerance in response to a nociceptive stimulus (radiant heat). Furthermore, there have been a number of reports concerning its efficacy in the management of pain from bony metastases and also in the treatment of 'cyclical' attacks of migraine; in these cases, an influence on serum prolactin levels must be considered important.

Bibliography

Battista, A. F. and Wolff, B. B. (1973). Levodopa and induced-pain response. *Arch. Intern. Med.*, **132,** 70

Behar, M., Magora, F., Olshwang, D. and Davidson, J. T. (1979). Epidural morphine in treatment of pain. *Lancet,* **1,** 527

Bourhis, A., Boudouresque, G., Pellet, W., Fondarai, J., Ponzio, J. and Spitalier, J. M. (1978). Pain infirmity and psychotropic drugs in oncology. *Pain,* **5,** 263

Bowman, W. C. and Rand, M. J. (1980). '*A Textbook of Pharmacology*'. (2nd edn.) (London and Oxford: Blackwell Scientific Publications)

Bresler, D. E. and Katz, R. L. (1980). 'Chronic pain: alternatives to neural blockade': In Cousins, M. J. and Bridenbaugh, P. O. (eds.) *Neural Blockade,* p. 651. (Philadelphia: J. B. Lippincott)

Budd, K. (1978). Psychotropic drugs in the treatment of chronic pain. *Anaesthesia,* **33,** 531

Clayman, C. B. (1975). The prostaglandins. *J. Am. Med. Assoc.,* **233,** 904

Cooper, J. R., Bloom, F. E. and Roth, R. H. (1978). *The Biochemical Basis of Neuropharmacology* (3rd edn.). (New York: Oxford University Press)

Eadie, M. J. and Tyrer, J. H. (1980). *Anticonvulsant Therapy. Pharmacological Basis and Practice.* 2nd edn. (Edinburgh: Churchill Livingstone)

Foldes, F. F. (1978). The role of drugs in the management of intractable pain. In Swerdlow, M. (ed.) *Relief of Intractable Pain.* 2nd edn. pp. 65–97 (Amsterdam: Excerpta Medica)

Halpern, L. M. (1977). Analgesic drugs in the management of pain. *Arch. Surg.,* **112,** 861

Halpern, L. M. (1979). Psychotropics, ataractics and related drugs. In: Bonica, J. J. and Ventafridda, V. (eds.) *Advances in Pain Research and Therapy II.* (New York: Raven Press)

Hatangdi, V. S., Boas, R. A., and Richards, D. G. (1976). Post herpetic neuralgia: management with antiepileptic & tricyclic drugs. In Bonica, J. J. and Ventavridda, V. (eds.) *Advances in Pain Research and Therapy I,* p. 583, (New York: Raven Press)

Houde, R. W. (1979). Role of analgesics and related drugs in visceral and perineal pain. In Bonica, J. J. and Ventrafridda, V. (eds.) pp. 589–591 *Advances in Pain Research and Therapy II.* (New York: Raven Press)

Houde, R. W. (1979). Systemic analgesics and related drugs: Narcotic analgesics. In Bonica, J. J. and Ventrafridda, V. (eds.) pp. 263–273 *Advances in Pain Research and Therapy II.* (New York: Raven Press)

Houde, R. W. (1979). Analgesic effect of the narcotic agonist-antagonist. *Br. J. Clin. Pharmacol.,* **7,** 2975

Howard, R. C., Milne, L. A. and Williams, N. E. (1980). Epidural morphine in terminal care. *Anaesthesia,* **35,** (In press)

Kocher, R. (1979). The use of psychotropic drugs in the treatment of cancer pain. In Bonica, J. J. and Ventafridda, V. (eds.) *Advances in Pain Research and Therapy II.* (New York: Raven Press)

Lee, R. and Spencer, P. S. J. (1977). Antidepressants and pain. *J. Int. Med. Res.,* **5,** 146

Lewis, J. W. and Rance, M. J. (1979). Opioids and the management of pain 2: Developments in therapy. *Pharmac. J.,* **222,** 61

Merskey, H. (1978). Psychological aspects of pain relief; hypnotherapy psychotropic drugs. In Swerdlow, M. (ed.) *Relief of Intractable Pain.* 2nd edn. pp. 21–48 (Amsterdam: Excerpta Medica)

Nathan, P. W. (1978). Chlorprothixene (Taractan) in post-herpetic neuralgia and other severe chronic pains. *Pain,* **5,** 367

Robbie, D. S. (1979). A trial of sublingual Buprenorphine in cancer pain. *Br. J. Clin. Pharmacol.* **7,** 3155

Ryan, W. G., Schwartz, T. B. and Perlia, C. P. (1969). Effect of Mithramycin on Paget's disease of Bone. *Trans. Assoc. Am. Phys.,* **82,** 353

Snyder, S. H. (1977). Opiate receptors in the brain. *N. Engl. J. Med.,* **296,** 266

Swerdlow, M. (1980). The treatment of 'shooting' pain. *Postgrad. Med. J.,* **56,** 159

Swerdlow, M. (1980). Anticonvulsants in the treatment of lancinating pains. *Proceedings of the 7th World Congress of Anaesthesiology.* (Amsterdam: Excerpta Medica) (In press)

Takemori, A. E. (1976). Pharmacologic factors which alter the action of narcotic analgesics and antagonists. *Ann. N. Y. Acad. Sci.,* **281,** 262

Turner, P. and Shand, D. G. (eds.) (1978). *Recent Advances in Clinical Pharmacology 1.* (Edinburgh: Churchill Livingstone)

Vane, J. K. (1976). The mode of action of aspirin and similar compounds. *J. Allergy Clin. Immunol.,* **58,** 691

Ware, S. B. and Millward-Sadler, G. H. (1980). Acute liver disease associated with sodium valproate. *Lancet,* **2,** 1110

Way, E. L. and Settle, A. A. (1975). Uses of narcotic antagonists. *Rational Drug Ther.,* **9,** 1

Williams, N. E. (1977). The role of drug therapy. In Lipton, S. (ed.) *Persistent Pain* Vol. 1. pp. 237–252 (London: Academic Press)

Wynne Aherne, E., Piall, E. and Twycross, R. G. (1979). Serum morphine concentration after oral administration of diamorphine hydrochloride and morphine sulphate. *Br. J. Clin. Pharmacol.,* **8,** 577

Yaksh, T. L. and Rudy, T. A. (1978). Narcotic analgetics. C.N.S. sites and mechanisms of action as revealed by intracerebral injection techniques. *Pain,* **4,** 299

5

Current views on the use of nerve blocking in the relief of chronic pain

A. S. Brown

INTRODUCTION

The universal accessibility of nerve blocking procedures, compared with the limited availability of specialized neurosurgical measures means that, in the present state of therapeutics, the former retain their wide acceptance and usefulness[1]. However, while they have a general usefulness, such blocks (and some neurosurgical procedures) are already being displaced in major pain relief centres by other forms of therapy. Temporary nerve blocks may be of value in confirming the differential diagnosis in some forms of chronic pain and occasionally produce more than temporary relief. Neurolytic agents can still provide a considerable degree of relief when properly employed, but when misused, complications may be serious or even fatal. The incidence of neuralgia and the recovery of sensation during the course of nerve regeneration make their use of more limited value in benign conditions.

NERVE BLOCKING TECHNIQUES

It is now generally agreed that if an area of denervation is to be produced or if sensory pathways are to be blocked neurolytically then preliminary local anaesthetic blocks should be carried out. If accurate nerve blocking techniques are used then the patient can be given some indication of the possible effect of the neurolytic block. Some may indeed prefer to retain pain, rather than lose all sensation; this applies with particular force to patients with trigeminal neuralgia.

Nerve blocking techniques are never a substitute for careful neurological assessment, but may be a useful adjunct to that examination[2]. However, under certain circumstances, differential sensory block produced by spinal or epidural anaesthesia may suggest that sensory blockade may be a useful form of therapy. Failure ultimately to achieve relief with localized blocks may throw doubt upon the validity of the diagnosis. Under these circumstances a temporary or only partial effect is produced unless very extensive, and usually unacceptable denervation is undertaken.

Nerve blocking techniques must be learned initially using local anaesthetic and only used for the injection of neurolytic agents when sufficient expertise has been gained. Somatic and visceral sensory innervation and the routing and distribution of the sensory, motor and automatic pathways must be known with precision otherwise interruption of the afferent or occasional motor pathway becomes a matter of chance. It is essential, therefore, that standard reference books on blocking procedures be available for consultation[3] [4]. Apart from their diagnostic value local anaesthetic blocks may produce relief of pain that lasts considerably longer than the local anaesthetic. As a test for accuracy of needle location, injection of a very small volume of procaine will produce immediate analgesia if it is deposited perineurally or is very close to the nerve. Many consider that this form of testing is now largely replaced by the small electrical nerve stimulator.

Clearly visceral afferent and efferent fibres (autonomic) and somatic sensory and motor fibres are accessible for interruption at the appropriate levels within the subarachnoid space, in the extradural space or paravertebrally where the spinal nerves exit through the intervertebral foraminae. Distal to this point somatic fibres with minimal autonomic representation may be blocked selectively in the course of the peripheral nerve. The autonomic (visceral) fibres can be blocked selectively in the sympathetic chain or other autonomic ganglia and plexuses.

Differences also exist in the intensity of the block that can be produced with the two major neurolytic agents. Alcohol is used to produce total neurolysis and should therefore completely interrupt conduction. Phenol, on the other hand, is used in a less destructive concentration to produce a so-called clinically selective block. Under these conditions strong stimulation will not be suppressed.

As with other forms of nerve section, neurolysis distal to the sensory root ganglion will be temporary until root regeneration occurs. Permanence will only occur if pre-ganglionic or ganglionic ablation is performed.

Nerve Blocking in the Relief of Chronic Pain

Kathleen M. Wood[5] introducing a comprehensive review on the use of phenol as a neurolytic agent observed that 'a patient with chronic intractable pain will often declare that he is willing to undergo anything to be free of his torment. The doctor who relieves him with a temporary nerve block may find the patient pleading for permanent interruption of the offending pain pathway. In this day of informed consent, one needs to know the possibilities of success, failure and especially of complications, so that both doctor and patient can make a rational decision'.

This advice must be carefully noted, for all procedures involving destruction of nerve tissue, particularly when using chemical neurolytic agents carry not only a risk of failure but also of potentially serious, and life endangering complications. That these dangers are not always understood, reported or fully discussed is perhaps reflected by the number of cases coming to litigation in the last few years. The dangers of using the various techniques involving phenol or chlorocresol may well limit their employment to the treatment of patients with malignant disease even though pain relief for other (non-malignant) conditions may be possible.

Early histopathological studies[6] proved conclusively that all neural elements are affected by phenol and that while there appeared to be a selective abolition of pain there was no selective destruction of neural material. Müller et al.[7] after comparative studies came to the conclusion that 3% aqueous solutions of phenol were as destructive on neural tissue as 40% alcohol. The mode of action of phenol as a neurolytic agent has been widely studied and was reviewed in 1974 by Felsenthal[8]. Burkel et al.[9] reported severe damage to the perineural vascular elements reaching their maximum effect within fourteen days. Nour-Eldin[10] noted a much greater affinity of phenol for aortic tissue than for neurophospholipid. This is consistent with the belief that phenol affects protein and could explain why many of the serious complications of phenol blocks are due to blood vessel damage.

After intrathecal injection phenol passes rapidly from the vehicle into solution in the CSF[11] and then spreads partly by diffusion through the spinal CSF and is absorbed into the blood stream. If spinal block or arachnoiditis is present, diffusion and dilution of the injected phenol is inhibited and excessively high concentrations build up leading to quite predictable but quite unnecessary serious neural damage and complications.

All neurolytic agents may cause a chemical neuritis of varying intensity and claimed to be between 2.0 and 10.0% of all administrations.

113

For convenience neurolytic procedures will be considered under the main headings of subarachnoid, subdural and extradural blocks, pituitary ablation, trigeminal ganglion block and peripheral nerve blocks (visceral and somatic).

Subarachnoid blocks

Absolute alcohol — posterior rhizotomy

Alcohol, being hypotonic, floats to the highest point of the dural sac. The patient is placed to position the roots to be blocked at the highest point of the spinal curve, subarachnoid puncture is performed adjacent to this and small fractions of alcohol injected until the desired effect is achieved[12]. Most workers restrict the procedure to one or two roots at a session. Complete permanent sensory loss is achieved. Alcohol destruction of anterior and posterior spinal roots or even spinal cord below the level of a complete physiological transection may be practiced occasionally in the management of seriously disabled paraplegic patients where uncontrollable involuntary muscle spasms are causing breakdown of skin from friction injuries or when rehabilitation and employment are being seriously compromised.

Spasticity and involuntary spinal movements have been treated and largely reported on by Nathan[19]. The concentration of neurolytic to achieve cessation of movement and release of spasticity is such that it leads to loss of cutaneous sensation and probably also to severe damage to other residual spinal cord functions. While such methods may be of value for a limited number of patients, if preservation of skin innervation is to be assured direct surgical exposure of the cord at laminectomy and anterior rhizotomy is the only certain approach.

Pain arising within non-functional damaged cord may also be treated by applying alcohol to the affected segment adjacent to the spinal block. This is a very limited and specialized application confined to patients within a paraplegic unit and its rehabilitation department, and will, therefore, not be considered further. Alcohol used in this way may avoid the need to perform extensive laminectomy and rhizotomies in seriously disabled patients.

In the author's experience alcohol has proved to be easier to control and to achieve satisfactory results than when phenol solutions were employed[13-15], possibly because of the difficulties of achieving a free flow of the viscid phenol solution in the presence of an arachnoiditis.

Phenol and chlorocresol

Phenol and chlorocresol subarachnoid blocks have gained widespread acceptance since the use of phenol was first reported by Maher[16] for the treatment of carcinoma pain. Alterations in techniques, variations in concentrations and constituents of the various solutions are well documented and will not be discussed[12,17,18,20-22]. Nathan reviewed the results of his twenty years experience in the treatment of pain and spasticity in 1972[19].

In the author's opinion the degree of blockade produced by agents other than alcohol is insufficient to obtund pain due to nerve entrapment between collapsing vertebral bodies or in severe spinal arthritic degeneration.

Techniques

Techniques of subarachnoid, extradural and subdural blocks are well documented in current literature[12,17,18,20]. The patient is placed in the postero-lateral decubitus with the roots to be blocked at the lowest point of the spinal curve. Subarachnoid puncture is made just cephalad to the highest root to be blocked. Once a free flow of CSF is obtained the chosen quantity of phenol glycerine solution is injected slowly to avoid mixing with CSF. The solution runs caudally lodging in the appropriate root pockets where it is concentrated producing its maximum effect on the sensory nerves at this point. If the procedure is carried out under X-ray control a small quantity of iophendlylate (Myodil) can be injected to try to visualize where the injectate will flow. Unfortunately the oily contrast medium can fill the desired root pockets and spread a protective layer of oil over the nerve protecting it from the action of the neurolytic. The only deviation from the generally accepted standard technique is that still used by the author when the total dose of phenol is divided into two equal fractions injected five minutes apart in an attempt to prolong the contact time between the neurolytic and nerve without subjecting the nerve to a higher initial concentration of phenol which would occur if a larger initial dose had been given. The author recommends a dose of 0.2 ml + 0.2 ml of 5% phenol for blocks at the L_5S_1 interval and increases the dose to 0.3 ml + 0.3 ml at $T_{12}L_1$ interval[21]. If there is any suggestion that the cauda equina has been entered by the needle, or if there is only an inadequate flow of CSF no attempt should be made to inject any neurolytic solution; such solution when injected into an encapsulated area where it cannot be diluted, will cause widespread and severe destruction.

Results of intrathecal phenol neurolysis from thirteen series of workers between 1958 and 1974 were analysed by Wood[5]. The results are difficult to analyse or compare. Few series reported poor results. Satisfactory results claimed by the majority varied between 77% and about 50%. The variations reported may have been due to a variety of causes. Initially selection may have been restricted to patients with a short life expectancy or to pain confined to the lower lumbar or sacral areas which are easier to deal with than lesions in the upper abdomen or thoraco-cervical regions. The few series included with poor results may have been due to inclusion of unsuitable patients or to a poor technique but this seems unlikely for their incidence of complications is not dissimilar to the more successful series, when due allowance is made for differences in pre-injection morbidity. When a partial sensory or motor loss is present before a neurolytic block is instituted, and this must mean that there is already loss of neural conductivity, the inevitable destruction caused by the neurolytic block must increase the extent and degree of the patient's disability.

Difficulties may arise when perineal pain is present because the fine roots of the cauda equina supplying the sphincters and detrusors of the bladder may be significantly damaged if too high a concentration of neurolytic agent is in contact with them. To overcome this Maher[22] believes that his technique of intrathecal drop will minimize the danger. Brown[21], however, considers that the dose recommended (0.6 ml phenol in glycerine) is still too high for safety and prefers to use two fractions of 0.1 ml of 5% phenol in glycerine given with an interval of 5 minutes between doses. He also believes that attempts at bilateral blocking at one session will contribute to impairment of bladder function to a greater degree than occurs when the two sides are blocked independently and about a week apart.

Extradural block
Satisfactory subarachnoid block can be consistently achieved up to about the level of D_6. Above this level the shape and capacity of the dorsal and cervical subarachnoid space make it difficult to localize and concentrate the small volume of phenol solution that can be safely used.

The author[21] believes that 1 ml of 7.5% phenol/glycerine solution deposited extradurally will produce complete relief of cancer pain in 45 to 50% of patients so treated and therefore prefers extradural block to subarachnoid block for all levels above D_6. Papo and Visca[20] commented on the poor results of using subarachnoid phenol above the mid-dorsal region and believe that extradural block is more satisfactory. Maher[23] also believes that epidural phenol block is superior to subarachnoid block in the cervical region. Lloyd[24], however, considers that epidural blocks are disappointing and have no place in the treatment of pain from malignant disease. Raftery[25] reports the satisfactory use of an aqueous solution of 6% phenol introduced by catheter in fractional doses into the cervical epidural space for the control of pain due to malignant disease. Although he finds it to be satisfactory and flexible he suggests that it might not be without risk. Extradural block presents no technical difficulties. Aqueous solutions have been employed (usually 6.0%) given in volumes of 5 ml or more and so have phenol/glycerine solutions (7.5% phenol in glycerine) for more localized use. The author prefers the latter and does not exceed 1 ml in volume blocking two or at most three sensory roots at a session. Others report the use of volumes of 3 ml or more.

Following the injection of phenol in glycerine into the extradural space, pain takes 5–10 minutes to disappear. During the next 48 hours or so attacks of severe lacinating pain may occur of sufficient intensity to require opiates for their relief. The attacks gradually fade and disappear after that time. Indications and contraindications for the use of extradural phenol are similar to those for the use of subarachnoid phenol.

A similar block can be carried out in the sacral canal using an aqueous phenol solution either introduced through the sacral hiatus when the sacral nerves are to be blocked or for more localized blocks through one of the sacral foraminae.

Subdural block

As an alternative to subarachnoid or extradural block Maher[26] proposed that subdural deposition of phenol in glycerine would allow better localization of the neurolytic solution. It can also be used in conjunction with the extradural blocking techniques. In the recently published proceedings of a symposium on the treatment of cancer pain, several contributors [27-32] have reviewed the development and current use of various neurolytic blocks of the somatic and visceral pathways. These results will not be considered in detail as they confirm the results of earlier publications of these almost universally accepted methods. The conclusions reached in the various sections also confirm the value of the currently accepted methods of treatment.

Intrathecal saline

This gives effects somewhat similar to those produced by subarachnoid or extradural phenol, relieving pain in a proportion of patients when pain is due to carcinoma but frequently for a much shorter time. Being administered in large volume (20 ml) problems associated with localizing small volumes as seen with phenol do not arise. It does not relieve incident pain or pain due to nerve entrapment.

Hitchcock[33] described the use of cold irrigation, but on reviewing his method he believed that he had used a hyperosmolar solution which gave lasting relief of pain and that cold probably had little effect. Hitchcock then abandoned cold hypertonic saline and reported the use of a single dose of 10 to 15% saline at room temperature, achieving satisfactory high blocks for patients with orofacial pain due to malignant disease[34].

Collins[35] discussed the result of treating twenty cases with partially frozen saline. He claimed excellent results in nine patients with causalgia, a good to excellent response for post herpetic neuralgia but only fair results for those with metastatic tumour and peripheral vascular disease. Tsubokawa's[36] results in ten patients including seven with metastatic tumours and one with phantom pain were not satisfactory for pain recurred within a week. Subsequent treatment gave further relief for only up to forty days.

Savitz and Malis[37] reported their experience of using irrigation of the spinal theca with isotonic iced saline at a temperature of between − 1 °C and 0 °C. Patients experienced severe paraesthesia and fasciculation of muscle during the period of cooling. Without light general anaesthesia the patient found the method unacceptable. Fasiculation stopped when cooling ceased but the unpleasant dysaesthasiae persisted for several hours. Of 26 patients treated 16 had carcinoma; only nine obtained complete relief from between eight days and eight months. Two patients with causalgia benefited but only for one month, while two with post herpetic and one with post thoracotomy neuralgia derived no relief.

Jewett and King[38] described a persistent conduction loss in monkey dorsal roots exposed to hypertonic saline and were able to demonstrate that this was due to the effect of hyperosmolar chloride ions. Cooling neither increased nor decreased the block. Hitchcock and Prandini[39] reviewed the result of treating 108 patients with intractable pain from malignant disease, as well as benign conditions. Results were not given in detail but it was claimed that over 50% of cancer patients still experienced reasonable pain relief until death supervened. Muscle weakness (3%) and sphincter disorders (8%) were the most important complications. One patient with pre-existing arachnoiditis and spinal block developed severe cauda equina damage attributed to the effect of hypertonic saline trapped round the cauda equina, below the level of the block where dilution with CSF could not take place.

Lucas *et al*[40] reviewed the results obtained from over 2000 patients treated with hypertonic saline. Their reported results confirm the claims of earlier reports on the value and complications of the method and of its limitations. In this series 11% had transient adverse reactions, but what were considered to be significant complications including paraplegia and quadriplegia occurred in about 1% of patients. Two deaths were included in his series.

The technique is simple but requires that the patient is anaesthetized because of the extreme discomfort, and reflex hyperventilation and hypertension that would otherwise distress the patient following injection. General anaesthesia does not block these reflex responses.

The patient is placed on the painful side and lumbar puncture is performed at L_3 or L_4/L_5 interval. Two or three ml of CSF are withdrawn for analysis and 20 ml of 10 to 15% sodium chloride at room temperature is rapidly injected. For pain in the lower part of the body the bed is given a 20° head up tilt whereas for pain in the upper part of the trunk the bed is tilted 20° head down. When bilateral pain is present the patient is placed on his back. Tachypnoea, tachycardia, fasiculation and hypertension develop rapidly. Anaesthesia is continued until fasiculation and tachypnoea cease, after half to three-quarters of an hour. If anaesthesia is discontinued earlier the patient complains bitterly of disagreeable paraesthesiae.

Because severe hypertension always occurs, patients with limited cardiovascular and respiratory reserve may be at risk from this technique, for the acute stress can occasionally precipitate acute cardiac failure. Such a pre-existing condition should therefore be considered a contraindication to the use of hypertonic saline intrathecal injection.

Subsequent experience by the author with this method for treatment of terminal cancer pain leads to the belief that this is probably not as useful, nor as satisfactory as phenol blocks for this purpose unless the patient is already in hospital and life expectancy is short. It seems more satisfactory to use phenol as a neurolytic blocking agent for localized pain, including visceral pain, or alcohol pituitary ablation even for a patient apparently in the terminal stages of disease. However, the use of potent analgesics such as phenazocine (Narphen) or buprenorphine given sublingually may be entirely satisfactory for ambulatory patients, without interfering with the patients' other daily activities.

In spite of these strictures a seriously ill terminal patient may gain complete relief from only one injection and the results may prove entirely adequate.

Barbotage

Although not employing a neurolytic agent barbotage must be mentioned. Barbotage was advocated by Lloyd and his associates[41] claiming that this relieved intractable pain of malignant disease for periods ranging from 2 days to 3 months. A Tuohy needle is placed in the lumbar theca and 10 ml of CSF is withdrawn. Barbotage is performed twenty to thirty times. Lack of further significant reports or corroborative evidence makes the method difficult to assess.

Pituitary ablation

Alcohol hypophysectomy

Control of pain for patients with diffuse metastatic neoplasia can be extremely difficult, because of its widespread nature. If pain cannot be abolished by conventional means, or specific therapy, or if the patient is not considered suitable for treatment by neurodestructive procedures (cordotomy, tractotomy etc.) then chemical hypophysectomy may be considered to be a more appropriate form of treatment than the use of strong analgesics.

Trans-sphenoidal hypophysectomy and implantation of yttrium by the same route are well established neurosurgical techniques. Chemical hypophysectomy for the control of cancer pain was first used by Moricca[42] in 1968 and by Hayward *et al.*[43] as an alternative to and following surgical pituitary ablation as a means of treating patients with hormone dependent tumours. Moricca inserts needles into the sella turcica by the transnasal approach under X-ray control. After entering the sphenoidal sinus and approaching the sella turcica the needle tip is directed to impinge on the posterior wall of the sella 2 mm below the top of the posterior clinoid process. Depending on the size of the sella more than one needle placement may be necessary. Once the needles are *in situ* small fractions of absolute alcohol (0.1 ml) are injected slowly to a total volume of 1 ml given over ten to fifteen minutes. His initial series was restricted to patients with hormone dependent tumours. Pain relief was almost always immediate and he believed it to occur too quickly to be brought about by hormonal change. He then extended the technique to patients with non-hormone dependent tumours. Between 1963 and 1973 Moricca treated 687 patients[42,44,45] with advanced, widespread malignant disease. He claimed relief of pain for 605, stating that relief was complete, immediate and lasting. It was necessary to repeat the procedure in a large proportion of cases on two occasions and occasionally on a third or fourth occasion. As would be expected there was a high incidence of diabetes insipidus which was easy to control with nasal administration of anti-diuretic hormone. Rhinorrhoea, diplopia and hemianopsia occurred throughout the series but were infrequent; percentage incidences were not given.

Miles and Lipton[46] believe that relief obtained in patients who are not hormone dependent could be the result of alcohol disrupting parts of the posterior hypothalamus, for they were able to demonstrate that in the cadaver a mixture of indian ink and iodophendylate (Myodil) spread through the hypothalamus and even into the third ventricle in five out of thirteen studies. In all, the material could be found in sections of hypothalamus. They postulate that the spread of alcohol within the hypothalamus might be the explanation for the relief of pain and cite Sano's work[47] on relieving pain by creating a discrete stereotactic lesion in the posterior hypothalamus. Careful surgical hypophysectomy relieves pain rapidly in patients with hormone dependent tumours possibly by rapid reduction in turbidity from changes in hormonal factors. Pain is not relieved, however, in patients with non-hormone dependent tumours as is seen after alcohol.

Lipton[48] believes that the technique is useful for widespread neoplasia but feels that the degree of relief is not as great as that produced by percutaneous cordotomy. He finds that 70% of his patients benefit initially; 40% are totally pain free for up to four months, but after that the percentage falls to 20%. The block is repeated when necessary. He reports complications due to the spread of alcohol to adjacent structures affecting minimally the optic nerve and chiasma and nearby cranial nerves. His mortality was 5% but details are not given. All his patients developed diabetes insipidus which was easily controlled by an anti-diuretic nasal spray. None of his patients showed regression of tumour.

Katz and Levin[49] reported a series of thirteen patients similarly treated, of whom eleven obtained marked symptomatic relief. Several showed considerable regression of tumour deposits, as did Moricca's patients, but not Lipton's. Complications noted were CSF leak from the needle tract and transient occular palsies. All had easily controlled diabetes insipidus. There were no deaths in the Katz and Levin series. While disagreeing with the explanation put forward by Miles and Lipton[46] that pain relief was due to the effect of alcohol on pain pathways within the hypothalamus or its connections with the periventricular or central grey matter, they were quite unable to offer an alternative hypothesis.

Madrid[50] reviewed the use of chemical hypophysectomy in 329 patients and claimed that complete pain relief was obtained in 67%, partial relief in 27% and no benefit in only 20 patients. He believes that the benefits of this technique, are its simplicity which allows it to be used in most general hospitals, within a normal X-ray department, and the reasonably high degree of success that can be achieved in patients whether the tumours are hormone or non-hormone dependent. The main complications in Madrid's report did not differ significantly from other series. There was a significant incidence of CSF leakage and rhinorrhoea (10%) and a small number of patients developed diplopia due to involvement of the occulomotor nerve by the neurolytic.

Trigeminal neurolysis

Undoubtedly the commonest reason for the destruction of the trigeminal ganglion and its preganglionic fibres, or occasionally of a division of the nerve is for the treatment of trigeminal neuralgia. Less frequently it may be used to abolish orofacial pain due to malignant disease. The introduction of carbamazepine (Tegretol) has markedly reduced the number of patients requiring trigeminal ablation but a significant number of patients do become refractory to medicinal therapy after about two years. Ablation of the individual branches of the trigeminal nerve may help briefly by abolishing the trigger zone, but will not relieve the patient of his trigeminal neuralgia. Such peripheral sections can rarely if ever be justified and should not be practiced. If the patient suffers from the condition described as 'central facial pain' caused by a lesion within the central nervous system which has been mistakenly diagnosed as trigeminal neuralgia, trigeminal ganglion ablation will only aggravate the patient's misery.

Alcohol ablation

The trigeminal ganglion lies in a fold of dura (Mekel's cave) on the wing of sphenoid in close association with the foramen ovale with its sensory root projecting backwards and in close association with its motor root. The three sensory divisions pass forward to supply the structures of the face and scalp. For ablative procedures the ganglion is most conveniently approached by the anterior approach (of Härtel[51]). The needle is passed through the foramen ovale where it is in close proximity to the ganglion and onwards for a few millimetres. Once CSF is encountered the needle tip is close to the sensory root. In a proportion of patients it may be possible to manipulate the needle so as to bring the tip in contact with selected fibres. Localization may be tested by injecting 0.1 ml of 0.5% procaine and if immediate anaesthesia develops in the desired area, the neurolytic agent can then be injected to destroy these fibres. It is not usually possible to be selective in all patients and destruction of the greater part of the nerve will result in anaesthesia in an extensive area of the trigeminal denervation. Once the needle tip is in the optimum position as shown by the results of injecting this very small quantity of local anaesthetic, fractions of 0.1 ml of absolute alcohol are injected until the desired effect is achieved. Up to 1 ml may be required. Should extra-occular palsies begin to develop injection is stopped until they pass, and the procedure is then reviewed. If anaesthesia is produced in the first or second divisions the patient must be warned of the risks of developing either corneal ulceration from unnoticed abrasion, or trophic ulceration of the nose. Both complications can be virtually prevented if excision of the superior cervical ganglion is carried out. Should ulceration occur healing will rapidly take place if sympathectomy is performed.

If malignant disease is the cause of pain its distribution will depend on the degree of invasion of the tumour. As long as it is confined to the trigeminal nerve distribution, alcohol ablation will be satisfactory. Once spread involves the glossopharyngeal nerve and branches or roots of the cervical plexus, neurolytic blocks for technical reasons will not provide satisfactory treatment. Treatment of the patient will then be either by surgical exposure and division of the trigeminal and glossopharyngeal sensory roots as they enter the brain stem along with division of the upper cervical posterior roots, if facilities are available, or alternatively, and less satisfactory, by the use of strong analgesics which may afford relief. A proportion of patients may benefit from alcohol pituitary adenolysis and this method should certainly be considered.

Phenol neurolysis
Jefferson[52] treated 37 patients using up to 0.5 ml of 5% phenol in glycerine. The needle is first inserted into the foramen ovale in the usual way and the patient is then placed in the sitting position so that the needle is vertical. Up to 0.5 ml in increments of 0.05–0.1 ml of 5% phenol in glycerine is injected until the desired effect is achieved. He reported good results for patients with trigeminal neuralgia, and little benefit for post herpetic neuralgia, but failed to achieve adequate levels of analgesia for the treatment of cancer pain. He reported only one complication. One patient developed a transient abducens nerve palsy. Jefferson made the point that it was possible with phenol to relieve trigeminal neuralgia without producing complete analgesia. This was in contrast to alcohol

which always produced dense anaesthesia. Mousel[53] reported 38 blocks yielding satisfactory results in 30 patients. Frothingham *et al.*[54] using the Jefferson technique treated twelve patients obtaining relief in nine, partial relief in two and no benefit in the last one. The Edinburgh group, using a similar technique, abandoned it because of recurrences occurring after 18 months to 2 years, but the immediate results were similar to the other series reported above.

Total sensory denervation as after trigeminal ganglion ablation may be followed, if the first division is affected, by a trophic or post-traumatic keratitis or, if the second division is involved, a trophic ulceration of the nose. Both yield to cervical sympathectomy and can be prevented by prophylactic excision of the superior cervical ganglion.

During the last few years, small, portable, high frequency lesion makers and stimulators have been developed suitable for both hospital and domiciliary use, and capable of producing easily controlled lesions in the root of the trigeminal nerve. It would appear that this form of sensory ablation has already completely replaced the use of chemical neurolytics in neurosurgical centres in many parts of the world and its use is expected to continue to spread.

Peripheral nerve blocks

The peripheral sensory and motor pathways can be interrupted at any convenient place along their distribution. By choice of a suitable technique the block can be largely confined to the somatic sensory fibres or to the visceral afferent and efferent pathways within the sympathetic chain, its ganglia and plexuses. Alternatively the rami communicantes may be blocked where they join the spinal roots at the intervertebral foraminae.

Coeliac plexus block

Moore[55] advocates the posterior approach to the coeliac ganglion where it overlaps the second lumbar vertebral body, using a bilateral posterolateral needle insertion. Each half of the ganglion is injected with 25 ml of a 50% solution of alcohol after ensuring that the needle is neither in the blood vessels nor subarachnoid space. Injection in the conscious patient causes severe upper abdominal burning pain of sufficient intensity that general anaesthesia must be used. Post-operatively there is also loss of vasomotor tone. Care must be exercised when the patient first sits up or becomes ambulatory for severe orthostatic hypotension may develop.

Gorbitz and Leavens[56] consider that Moore's blind approach is unsatisfactory and recommend placing two Teflon catheters, one into each side of the coeliac plexus and adjusting their position until full pain relief can be achieved by a single injection of 5 ml of 1% lignocaine. Once this is established it is followed by an injection of 25 ml of 25% alcohol into each half of the plexus. They believe that X-ray control is necessary for satisfactory results. The results from both methods of treating upper abdominal pain or pain from pancreatitis appear to be comparable. In practice, considerably smaller volumes of either alcohol or phenol solution are adequate for most patients; for thin, emaciated individuals, 12.5 ml on each side will suffice. Apart from loss of vasomotor control that can persist for some time, alcohol neuritis remains a significant complication possibly affecting up to 15% of patients treated. However, the incidence varies widely and depends on spread of alcohol to effect adjacent sensory nerve fibres. No deaths have been reported in the recent literature.

A technique for blocking the coeliac plexus and the presacral nerves using 6% phenol similar to that already considered under alcohol blocks is also in use. The effect is similar to that produced by alcohol[56], but unlike the latter the injection is painless. Studies by Nour-Eldin[10] suggest that phenol is more likely to induce thrombosis than alcohol and this danger must be taken seriously. Because of the risk of vascular thrombosis, a risk well recognized by previous generations of vascular surgeons, phenol should probably not be used for blocks of the abdominal visceral sympathetic plexuses. A 50% solution of alcohol is as effective as phenol for this purpose but does not appear to be significantly thrombogenic.

Sympathectomy

Reid[57] described a technique of chemical *lumbar sympathectomy*. Fyfe and Quin[58] using a similar technique showed that while sympathetic block improved blood flow and temperature in superficial tissues it had no beneficial effect on intermittent claudication. Intermittent claudication does not yield to phenol block although resting pain is controlled.

Hughes-Davies and Redman[59] reported their experience of 124 blocks. The accuracy of their needle placement was confirmed by X-ray control. Ninety-seven patients with distal ischaemia due to atherosclerosis had chemical lumbar sympathectomy performed. All complained of rest pain associated with foot ischaemia or incipient gangrene. Needles were placed and injection made at the level of L_3 and L_4 bodies using the technique described by Reid[57]. Four ml of 6% phenol in water, was injected through each needle. There were 85 clinically helpful blocks and 39 classified as useless. They believed that the relief of rest pain, the feeling of warmth in the previously cold limb and reversal of pre-gangrenous skin changes were the major benefits. Some patients could walk more comfortably; however, intermittent claudication was not helped.

Block of the visceral afferent and efferent pathways to the lower limbs may be performed peripherally within the body of psoas where it lies paravertebrally. Feldman and Yeung[60] carried out paravertebral somatic blocks using 7.5% phenol in iophendylate (Myodil) for the treatment of vascular insufficiency of the lower limbs. Needles are inserted lateral to L_2 body and lie in psoas muscle. Five to 10 ml of solution are injected under X-ray control. The solution is confined within the muscle sheath. Twenty-eight patients were treated and immediate relief occurred in 90% of them; after 1 year 85% were still satisfactory. A painful neuritis lasting for 2 months occurred in two patients.

Temporary relief can be obtained by inducing a sympathectomized state in the lower limbs by retrograde intravenous infusion of guanethidine. The response to guanethidine can be used as a possible indicator for the possible later induction of lumbar sympathectomy[61]. Such a block is usually effective for about a week.

Post traumatic sympathetic dystrophy
In a considerable proportion of patients this yields to repeated sympathetic blocks with 2% lignocaine or other local anaesthetic. Carron and Weller[62] reported a failure rate of only six out of 108 patients studied. Those with upper limb involvement received a block of the stellate ganglion with 2% lignocaine on alternate days for five treatments. Lower limb pain was treated similarly, block being performed at the L_2 ganglion.

Peripheral somatic blocks
These can be performed where the nerve lies in an accessible position. Blocking is performed using a 6% aqueous solution of phenol. Both cervical and brachial plexuses are accessible for neurolytic blocking if this can be justified. The roots of the two plexuses emerge between the transverse process of the cervical and upper thoracic vertebrae and if the neurolytic solution is deposited at the tip of the transverse processes it will block the roots as they emerge. Block of the cervical plexus is easy to achieve when orofacial pain extends into the cervical distribution. Five ml of 5% aqueous phenol is deposited around the anterolateral portion of the cervical transverse processes. One root is blocked at each level. Any

motor loss is inconsequential if the block is correctly done. Neither vagus and phrenic nerves nor the carotid sheath should be implicated or compromised.

If the brachial plexus is involved in tumour or caught up in fibrous tissue local neurolytic blocks are quite inadequate. Movement of the upper limb or head and neck puts traction on the plexus, roots, and spinal cord and the degree of stimulus is such that severe pain continues to be generated. Rest pain, however, may be abolished. A similar approach to that used for cervical plexus block to reach the lateral aspect of the transverse processes may be possible depending on the extent of the tumour. A 2.5 to 3% aqueous solution of phenol will usually abolish resting pain and preserve a useful degree of motor function in a reasonable number of patients, but for worthwhile relief under the condition envisaged high cervical cordotomy or higher tractotomies offer the only reasonable prospect of satisfactory pain relief.

As with all other peripheral nerve blocks, neuritis is a major complication in 2 to 10% of patients and may be as distressing as the condition it was proposed to treat. When it occurs it may be considerably more difficult to manage.

Complications of neurolytic blocks

Many are listed in the literature. Some other blocks may produce partial loss of function which may be fully anticipated when there is already prior evidence of partial sensory or motor loss due to disease. Such a predictable outcome can hardly be reasonably classed as a complication in the sense of it being misadventure. Motor or sensory loss may follow the injection of excessive volumes or concentrations of neurolytic agents in an endeavour finally to relieve pain that is proving refractory, instead of using alternative forms of treatment.

Major loss of sensory and motor function can also be anticipated if the neurolytic solution is injected into an encapsulated area within the spinal theca, below a spinal block or within a matted and slightly adherent cauda equina.

Apart from technical disasters the danger of *thrombosis* arising after the injection of phenol solution remains a grave although fortunately infrequently reported hazard. The number of cases reported probably do not represent more than a fraction of those that occur.

Hughes[63] described a patient with a malignant stricture of the oesophagus treated by an intrathecal block at $T_{3,4}$, using 1 ml of 5% phenol in glycerine. Spastic paraparesis developed but recovered almost completely within ten days. The patient died seven weeks later and at autopsy there was a limited area of spinal cord infarction in association with thrombosis of branches of the posterior spinal artery at the level of the phenol block.

Superville–Sovak et al.[64] reported a more extensive vascular lesion after performing a cervical subdural block with 3 ml of 5% phenol in glycerine. The patient required ventilation until death after five weeks. At autopsy there was extensive intimal damage of small arteries on the surface of the nerve roots and under the lower surface of the cerebellum which also showed small areas of infarction.

Holland and Yousef[65] described a similar picture following a cervical subarachnoid injection of 6% phenol in glycerine using Maher's technique[22]. One ml of solution was injected followed over 5 minutes by four fractions of 0.5 ml. Apnoea developed shortly after and the patient was ventilated until death supervened some weeks later.

Totoki et al.[66] also reported a thrombosis of the anterior spinal artery after the injection of 0.3 ml of 10% phenol glycerine solution into the subarachnoid space at $C_{4.5}$ level. Respiratory failure required mechanical ventilation for 25 days. The initial flaccid quadriplegia progressed into a spastic paralysis. Death occurred at four months. The spinal cord showed loss of structure in the area of supply of the anterior spinal artery and areas of demyelination involving other areas of the cord examined at the level of the block.

The author has been consulted twice in the last five years about two patients who died following massive coeliac artery thrombosis and inferior mesenteric artery thrombosis following phenol sympathectomy procured with 6% aqueous solution of phenol. Neither case was reported.

Finally high concentrations of phenol–glycerine solution are extremely destructive. A case is reported in the annual report of the Medical Defence Union for 1979 of a surgeon who injected 1 ml of 10% phenol in glycerine into the lumbar subarachnoid space to treat pain associated with failed surgery for back pain. The patient was left with marked sensory loss and loss of bladder function.

In each major complication several factors seem to operate. A high concentration of the neurolytic is severely destructive, as is a normal dose injected into an encysted area of the subarachnoid space. When extradural or high subarachnoid blocks are performed in the presence of pre-existing interference with the anterior or posterior spinal arteries, as would be present for example in a spondylitic spine, this pathology may provide the focus for the subsequent development of a spreading infarction due to thrombosis, a factor that operated in several of the above cases.

Hypertonic saline has not been implicated in delayed spinal cord thrombosis but on several occasions severe cervical and medullary transient disturbances have been reported but all resolved almost completely in 3 to 4 days. All were associated with attempts at very high blocks.

Several patients have developed paraplegia or quadriplegia which in some instances was certainly due to the injection of hypertonic saline into the subarachnoid space below a complete spinal block preventing dilution of the injectate. The result of such a misadventure can certainly be anticipated for this is similar to the results following other neurolytics under the same circumstances.

Denervation dysaesthesiae
This consists of a variety of conditions including post herpetic neuralgia, central pain arising from spinal cord injury or disease, and certain neuropathies among others, all characterized by a considerable reduction in sensory input to spinal cord. Some, such as post herpetic neuralgia, undergo complete final remission: others, such as those resulting from trauma will persist. Careful clinical examination always shows a varying degree of sensory loss which may be partly obscured by a cutaneous dysaesthesia.

Extensive so-called sensory diagnostic blocks, especially if differential spinal or epidural or sympathetic blocks are used will suggest that pain can be relieved by definitive neurolysis. However, if neurolysis, chemical or surgical, is carried out, pain returns within a few days and the patient is then worse off than before due to further sensory deprivation. As a corollary, increasing the sensory input to the cord by transcutaneous stimulation if sufficient cutaneous stimulation is possible, or direct dorsal column stimulation if absent is usually effective.

Pain arising within the spinal cord as the result of trauma or damage from tumour and secondary paraplegia may occasionally be treated by alcohol destruction of the affected segment of cord, provided the patient can tolerate the upward extension of his already severe spinal cord defect.

The use of ablation procedures for the denervation dysaesthesiae, however attractive this may initially appear, should be firmly avoided, other methods of therapy being of greater benefit.

Non-neurolytic methods
Many benign conditions causing chronic pain are not amenable to treatment with neurolytic substances, in part because of the short duration of

action of these substances, or because of the nature or site of the lesion.

Chronic backache has been treated for the last forty years in many ways including sacral and lumbar epidural injections of physiological saline or local anaesthetic, with or without manipulation. Steroids were added to these solutions in the early 1950s.

Few series of reports give any adequate pathological or clinical details, but each probably represents a considerable heterogeneous collection of varying pathologies. Comparison of series or even methods employed within one are difficult. Warr *et al.*[67] treated a series of patients with lumbar disc derangement, spondylosis and spondylolisthesis and those who had a recurrence of symptoms after laminectomy. They injected epidurally a mixture of 40 ml of 0.75% lignocaine to which they added 80 mg of methylprednisolone and 25 mg of hydrocortisone. They believed that the large volume injected would help separate minor adhesions. After injection spinal manipulation was carried out. Of 500 patients treated 317 benefited.

Winnie and Ramamurthy[68] believed that although steroids applied locally within the epidural space resulted in marked relief of pain particularly when associated with an inflammatory reaction and arachnoiditis, the intrathecal route had no advantage. Previous reports[69,70] had suggested that the subarachnoid route might be more suitable.

Forrest[71] used epidural steroids in the cervical and thoracic as well as lumbar regions for a variety of syndromes. His technique differed from the usually accepted large volume of others in this field. Small volumes of concentrated solutions were deposited at the level of the nerve roots involved by individual needle placement. For multi-level blocks a separate needle insertion was made for each root to be treated and a similar volume of solution was deposited at each. One week later and at weekly intervals for three blocking sessions this was repeated. Forrest reported that 86% of patients with post herpetic neuralgia were pain free after 6 months, but this has not been found universally in patients with chronically established neuralgia. Patients with post surgical and post traumatic pain benefited much less, only 40% being free of pain one month after their third and last injection. The side effects of steroid therapy in this series were reported as a slight gain in weight, and slight rise in blood pressure, both of which resolved spontaneously.

James and Little[72] treated 50 patients with chronic benign hip pain mostly with osteoarthritis or associated with muscle spasm. Local anaesthetic blocks using 0.5% bupivacaine of the obturator nerve and the nerve to quadratus femoris are performed percutaneously. Many patients had worthwhile relief which they attributed to the local anaesthetic breaking the cycle of pain/spasm/pain. They felt that a course of blocks might be indicated for some of these patients.

Similar local anaesthetic solutions can be used for nerve blocking or more frequently local infiltration, of tender areas of muscle associated with local spasm which yield in many instances to repeated blocks associated with physiotherapy when the local anaesthetic action allows painless manipulation of the myalgic spots. Bourne[73] described the use of local infiltration with 2 ml of 1% lignocaine containing 10 mg of triamcinalone, which is an antifibrinolytic unsuitable for repeated injection. He claimed satisfactory results for the majority of his patients, and considers that the use of such an antifibrinolytic might be of value in treating chronic backache associated with myalgia.

Diagnostic blocks

It has been not uncommon for anaesthetists and others to use local anaesthetic blocking techniques as a diagnostic tool to supplement neurological assessment[17,69,72]. Apart from blocking being carried out for diagnostic assessment the patient is given the opportunity of experiencing what the result of sensory blockade would feel like and to decide perhaps on several occasions whether the result would be acceptable or not, before having the definitive permanent block carried out.

References

1 Swerdlow, M. (1979). Subarachnoid and extradural neurolytic blocks. In Bonica, J. J., and Ventafridda, V. (eds). *Advances in Pain Research and Therapy.* Vol. 2 p. 325. (New York: Raven Press)
2 Bonica, J. J. (1974). Current Role of Nerve Blocks in Diagnosis and Therapy of Pain. In Bonica, J. J., (ed). *Advances in Neurology,* Vol. 4 (New York: Raven Press)
3 Pitkin, G. P. *Conduction Anaesthesia.* 2nd Edn. (Philadelphia: Lippincott)
4 Eriksson, E. (ed). (1979). *Illustrated Handbook of Local Anaesthesia* (Copenhagen: I. C. Sorenson)
5 Wood, K. M. (1978). Use of phenol as a neurolytic agent: a review. *Pain,* **5,** 205
6 Smith, M. C. (1964). Histological findings following intrathecal injection of phenol solutions for the relief of pain. *Br. J. Anaesth.,* **36,** 387
7 Möller, J. E., Holweg-Larsen, J. and Jacobsen, E. (1969). Histopathological lesions in sciatic nerve of the rat following perineural application of phenol and alcohol solution. *Dan. Med. Bull.,* **16,** 116
8 Felsenthal, G. (1974) Pharmacology of phenol in peripheral nerve block: a review. *Arch. Phys. Med. Rehab.,* **55,** 13
9 Burkel, W.E. and McPhee, M. (1970). Effect of phenol injection into peripheral nerve of the rat. Electron microscope studies. *Arch. Phys. Med. Rehab.,* **51,** 391

10 Nour-Eldin, F. (1970). Preliminary report: uptake of phenol by vascular and brain tissue. *Microvasc. Res.,* **2,** 224

11 Ichiyanagi, K., Matsuki, M., Kenefuchi, S . and Kato, Y. (1975). Progressive changes in the concentration of phenol and glycerine in the human subarachnoid space. *Anaesthesiology,* **42,** 622

12 Lipton, S. (1979). The control of pain (*Current Topics in Anaesthesia – 2*) (London: Edward Arnold)

13 Dimitrijevic, M.R. and Nathan, P.W. (1967). Studies of spasticity in man. 1. Some features of spasticity. *Brain,* **90,** 1

14 Churcher, M. (1978). Peripheral nerve blocks in relief of intractable pain. In Swerdlow, M. (ed.) *Relief of Intractable Pain,* 2nd Edn. pp. 99–120 (Amsterdam: Experta Medica)

15 Papo, I. and Visca, A. (1976). Intrathecal phenol in the treatment of pain and spasticity. *Progress in Neurological Survey,* **7,** 56

16 Maher, R. M. (1955). Relief of pain in incurable cancer. *Lancet,* **1,** 18

17 Bonica, J. J. (1953). *The Management of Pain.* (Philadelphia: Lea and Febiger)

18 Swerdlow, M. (1978). In Swerdlow, M. (ed.). *Relief of Intractable Pain,* 2nd Edn. pp. 121–155 (Amsterdam: Excerpta Medica)

19 Nathan, P. W. (1972). Pain in cancer. Comparison of results of cordotomy and chemical rhizotomy. In Fusek, J. and Kung, Z. (eds.) *Present Limits of Neurosurgery,* p. 513. (Amsterdam: Excerpta Medica)

20 Papo, J. and Visca, A. (1974). Phenol rhizotomy in the treatment of cancer pain. *Anaesth. Analg.,* **53,** 993

21 Brown, A. S. (1961). Treatment of intractable pain by nerve block with phenol. Excerpta Medica. *Int. Congress Series,* **36,** E.59

22 Maher, R. M. and Mehta, M. (1977). Spinal intrathecal and extradural analgesia. In Lipton, S. (ed.) *Persistent Pain,* Chap. 4. (London and New York: Academic Press)

23 Maher, R. M. (1966). Phenol for pain and spasticity. In *Pain* Harry Ford Hospital International Symposium. (New York: Little, Brown)

24 Lloyd, J. W. (1976). Practical regional analgesia. In Lee, J. A. and Bryce Smith, R. (eds.) *Monograph in Anaesthesiology,* p. 216. (New York: American Elsevier)

25 Raftery, H. (1977). Extradural injection of 5% aqueous solution of phenol for cervical pain. Presented at meeting of *Intractable Pain Society of Great Britain*

26 Maher, R. M. (1960). Further experience with intrathecal and subdural phenol. Observations on two forms of pain. *Lancet,* **1,** 895

27 Papo, I. and Visca, A. (1979). Phenol rhizotomy for the treatment of cancer pain – a personal account of 290 cases. In Bonica, J. J. and Ventafridda, V. (eds.) *Advances in Pain Research and Therapy,* Vol. 2, pp. 339–346 (New York: Raven Press)

28 Madrid, J. L. and Bonica, J. J. (1979). Cranial nerve blocks. In Bonica, J. J. and Ventafridda (eds.) *Advances in Pain Research and Therapy,* Vol. 2 pp. 347–355 (New York: Raven Press)

29 Swerdlow, M. (1979). Role of nerve blocks in pain involving the chest and brachial plexus. In Bonica, J. J. and Ventafridda, V. (eds.). *Advances in Pain Research and Therapy,* Vol. 2, pp. 567–576 (New York: Raven Press)

30 Moore, D. C. (1979). Role of nerve block and neurolytic solutions in visceral and perineal pain. In Bonica, J. J. and Ventafridda, V. (eds.) *Advances in Pain Research and Therapy,* Vol. 2, pp. 593–596 (New York: Raven Press)

31 Ventafridda, V. (1979). Neurolytic block in perineal pain. In Bonica, J. J. and Ventafridda, V. (eds.) *Advances in Pain Research and Therapy,* Vol. 2, p. 597. (New York: Raven Press)

32 Bonica, J. J. and Ventafridda, V. (eds.) (1979). *Advances in Pain Research and Therapy,* Vol. 2, pp. 597–603 (New York: Raven Press)

33 Hitchcock, E. R. (1967). Hypothermic subarachnoid irrigation. *Lancet*, **1**, 434

34 Hitchcock, E. R. (1969). Osmolytic neurolysis for intractable facial pain. *Lancet*, **1**, 434

35 Collins, J. R., Juras, E. P. and van Hourten, R. J. (1969). Intrathecal cold saline solution. A new approach to pain. *Anaesth. Analg.*, **48**, 816

36 Tsubokawa, T. (1969). Method for pain relief by injection of frozen physiological saline into the spinal subarachnoid space. Clinical results. *Brain Nerve*, Tokyo, **21**, 693

37 Savitz, M. H. and Malis, L. I. (1972). Intrathecal injection of isotonic iced saline for intractable pain. *Mount Sinai J. Med.*, **34**, 134

38 Jewett, D. L. and King, J. S. (1971). Conduction block of monkey dorsal rootlets by water and hypertonic solutions. *Exp. Neurol.*, **33**, 225

39 Hitchcock, E. R. and Prandini, M. N. (1973). Hypertonic saline in the management of intractable pain. *Lancet*, **1**, 310

40 Lucas, J. T., Ducker, T. B. and Perot, P. L. (1975). Adverse reactions to intrathecal saline injection for control of pain. *J. Neurosurg.*, **42**, 557

41 Lloyd, J. W., Hughes, J. T. and Davies-Jones, G. A. B. (1972). Relief of severe intractable pain by babotage of the cerebro-spinal fluid. *Lancet*, **1**, 354

42 Moricca, G. (1968). *Progress in Anaesthesiology*, In *Proceedings of Fourth World Congress of Anaesthesiologists* (Amsterdam: Excerpta Medica)

43 Hayward, T. L., Atkins, H. T. B., Falconer, M. A., MacLean, K. S., Salman, L. F. W., Schurr, P. H. and Shaheen, C. H. (1970). Clinical trials comparing transfrontal hypophysectomy with adrenalectomy and transethmoidal hypophysectomy. In Joslin, C. A. F. and Gleave, E. N. (eds.) *Clinical Management of Advanced Breast Cancer* (Cardiff: Alpha Omega Alpha)

44 Moricca, G. (1974). Chemical hypophysectomy for cancer pain. In Bonica, J. J. (ed.) *Advances in Neurology* Vol. 4, p. 707. (New York: Raven Press)

45 Moricca, G. (1976). Neuroadenolysis (Chemical hypophysectomy) for diffuse unbearable cancer pain. In Bonica, J. J. and Albe-Fessard, D. (eds.) *Advance in Pain Research and Therapy*, Vol. 1, p. 863. (New York: Raven Press)

46 Miles, J. and Lipton, S. (1976). The mode of action by which pituitary alcohol injection relieves pain. In Bonica, J. J. and Albe-Fessard, D. (eds.) *Advances in Pain Research*, Vol. 1, pp. 867–869 (New York: Raven Press)

47 Sano, K. (1973). Presented at Symposium Sur la Doleur, Paris

48 Lipton, S. (1978). Pituitary injection of alcohol. In *Control of Chronic Pain* (Current topics in anaesthesia–2) pp. 104–107 (London: Edward Arnold)

49 Katz, J. and Levin, A. B. (1977). Treatment of diffuse metastatic cancer pain by instillation of alcohol into the Sella Turcica. *Anaesthesiology*, **46**, 115

50 Madrid, J. L. (1979). Chemical hypophysectomy. In Bonica, J. J. and Ventafridda, V. (eds.) *Advances in Pain Research and Therapy*, Vol. 2, pp. 381–391 (New York: Raven Press)

51 Härtel, F. (1920) *Die Lakalanestherie*, p. 120 (Stuttgart: Ferdinand Enke)

52 Jefferson, A. (1963). Trigeminal root and ganglion injections using phenol in glycerine for the relief of trigeminal neuralgia. *J. Neurol. Neurosurg. Psychiatr.*, **26**, 345

53 Mousel, L. H. (1967). Treatment of intractable pain of the head and neck. *Anaesth. Analg.*, **46**, 705

54 Frothingham, R. E., Atchison, J. W. D. and Bailey, C. C. (1974). Treatment of facial pain by percutaneous injection of the gasserian ganglion. *T.S.C. Med. Assoc.*, **70**, 1960

55 Moore, D. C. (1979). Coeliac (spanchnic) plexus block with alcohol for cancer pain of upper intra abdominal viscera. In Bonica, J. J. and Ventafridda, V. (eds.) *Advances in Pain Research and Therapy*, Vol. 2, p. 357 (New York: Raven Press)

56 Gorbitz, C. and Leavens, M. E. (1971). Alcohol block of the coeliac plexus for control of upper abdominal pain caused by cancer and pancreatitis. *J. Neurosurg.*, **34**, 575

57 Reid, W., Watt, J. K. and Gray, T. G. (1970). Phenol injection of the sympathetic chain. *Br. J. Surgery*, **57**, 45

58 Fife, T. and Quin, R. D. (1975). Phenol sympathectomy in the treatment of intermittent claudication: a controlled clinical trial. *Br. J. Surg.*, **62**, 68

59 Hughes-Davies, D. I. and Rechman, L. R. (1976). Clinical lumber sympathectomy. *Anaesthesia*, **31**, 1068

60 Feldman, S. A. and Yeung, M. L. (1975). Treatment of intermittent claudication. Lumbar paravertebral somatic block with phenol. *Anaesthesia*, **30**, 174

61 Hannington-Kiff, J. G. (1974). Intravenous regional sympathetic block. In Hannington-Kiff, J. G. (ed.) *Pain Relief*, p. 69. (London: Heinemann Medical)

62 Carron, H. and Weller, R. M. (1974). Treatment of post traumatic sympathetic dsytrophy. In Bonica, J. J. (ed.) *Advances in Neurology 4*, pp. 485-490, (New York: Raven Press)

63 Hughes, J. T. (1970). Thrombosis of posterior spinal artery. *Neurology*, **20**, 659

64 Superville-Savak, B., Rasmusky, M. and Finlayson, M. H. (1975). Complications of phenol neurolyses. *Arch. Neurol.*, **32**, 226

65 Holland, A. J. C. and Yousef, M. (1978). A complication of subarachnoid phenol blockade. *Anaesthesia*, **34**, 260

66 Totoki, T., Kato, T., Nomoto, Y., Kurakazu, M. and Kamasahi, T. (1979). Anterior spinal syndrome as a complication of cervical intrathecal injection. *Pain*, **6**, 99

67 Warr, A. C., Wilkinson, J. A., Burn, J. M. B. and Langdon, L. (1972). Chronic lumbo-sacral syndrome treated by epidural injection and manipulation. *Practitioner*, **209**, 53

68 Winnie, A. P. and Ramamurthy, S. (1976). Steroid for discogenic pain. In *Proc. VI World Congress of Anaesthesiology*. Abstract. (New York: American Elsevier)

69 Winnie, A. P. and Collins, V. J. (1968). The pain clinic I: Differential neural blockade in pain syndromes of questionable etiology. *Med. Clin. N. Am.*, **52**, 1968

70 Winnie, A. P., Hartman, J. T. and Meyers, H. L., jun. (1972). The pain clinic II: Intradural and extradural corticosteroids for sciatica. *Anaesth. Analg. (Cleve)*, **51**, 990

71 Forrest, J. B. (1978). Management of chronic dorsal root pain with epidural steroid. *Canad. Anesth. Soc. J.*, **25**, 218

72 James, C. D. T. and Little, T. F. (1976). A simplified technique for the relief of intractable osteoarthritic pain. *Anaesthesia*, **31**, 1060

73 Bourne, I. H. J. (1979). Treatment of backache with local injection. *Practitioner*, **222**, 708

74 Winnie, A. P., Ramamurthy, S. and Durravi, Z. (1974). Diagnostic and therapeutic nerve blocks. Recent advances in techniques. In Bonica, J. J. (ed.) *Advances in Neurology*, Vol. 4, pp. 455–460 (New York: Raven Press)

6

Current views on the role of neurosurgery for pain relief

E. Hitchcock

INTRODUCTION

There has recently been a gradual re-awakening of the interest of neuro-surgeons in the management of intractable pain. With notable exceptions neurosurgical involvement declined during the period when the only effective treatment for intractable pain appeared to be two simple and well established techniques; cordotomy and retrogasserian trigeminal rhizotomy. Even these were not without complications and it is possible that advances in other techniques, such as microsurgery, attracted attention away from what must often have seemed unrewarding exercises. The tendency for pain recurrence was often viewed as inevitable and the development of new procedures viewed against a background of therapeutic nihilism. Much of this depression was related to the concept of 'pain pathways'. Earlier generations had felt secure in performing sections and re-sections based on the anatomical and physiological knowledge available at that time. Gradually experience showed that these pathways were less clearly defined and less dominant than had been expected. Keller[1] summarizing the development of our concepts of central pathways concluded that the evidence indicated that central pain pathways include both neo- and paleospinothalamic systems as well as the brain stem reticular formation. One of the most intractable pain syndromes is central pain and Cassinari and Pagni[2] reviewing the evidence presented a strong case for invoking polysynaptic systems as the cause. Over the past decade therefore much attention has been given to produc-

135

ing lesions in various parts of this system with varying degrees of success. The encouragement given by research into the development of new procedures is reflected in the rise and fall of particular techniques as support for novel neurophysiological concepts waxes and wanes.

There is a clear tendency to replace the older open operations with percutaneous and stereotactic procedures as their obvious advantages became more widely appreciated. Apart from their value in frail patients unsuitable for general anaesthesia, hospitalization is short and complications fewer. Their success in producing longlasting pain relief compared to open procedures is still debatable however. Against the advantage of precise physiological localization by stimulation in the conscious patient instead of direct anatomical visualization in the anaesthetized patient is the disadvantage of 'physiological' lesions which may recover. Transient sensory changes are commoner after percutaneous operations than open sections encouraging many surgeons to reserve the former for patients with terminal disease. The advantage of electrical stimulation in identification of targets has also encouraged radiofrequency destruction rather than chemical lysis which is poorly localized. Not all patients are prepared to submit to procedures under local anaesthesia, however, and the requirement of general anaesthesia makes percutaneous analgesic procedures difficult or impossible.

The welcome addition of basic scientists to the study of human pain has encouraged reconsideration of the purpose and mechanism of many operations but physiologists in particular have not hesitated to criticize on practical grounds procedures such as rhizotomy and cordotomy. A brief perusal of selected clinical literature has produced a number of statements based on small and inaccurate evidence which questions the value of procedures known to be effective. A small series of thoracic cordotomies performed by different surgeons of varying experience[3] is often quoted as revealing a high rate of recurrence and used as an argument against the procedure. Other larger and individual series[4] have provided contrary evidence for it is clear that poor results are largely due to poor patient selection and incomplete incision.

For all surgical analgesia the choice must be guided by three important principles.

(1) The procedure should not incapacitate the patient.
(2) The sensory loss should cover any anticipated extension of pain (c.f. malignancy).
(3) Relief should be complete and long lasting.

Procedures with high mortality or morbidity must be critically examined therefore, especially for patients with pain due to benign disease. An early surgical referral is most important so that definitive procedures can be performed before static pain patterns develop and before the inevitable psychological accompaniments of severe pain became predominant. Regrettably many patients are referred for analgesic surgery in poor general condition which restricts the choice of procedure. Because of this many surgical procedures have developed which can be used in this common group of patients.

Although a vast variety of painful syndromes are referred for pain relief one of the commonest causes and one requiring urgent intervention is pain due to malignancy. Even here the influence of mind is often apparent and surgical success is often related to astute assessment and management of accompanying behaviour. The widespread acceptance of the importance of the emotional state in pain syndromes has encouraged much work on the psychological assessment of pain states (Figure 1) and an increasing tendency to explore non-surgical methods. Many reports have appeared from clinics that appear to be managed without the benefit of neurological or neurosurgical advice and such reports frequently reveal bias or ignorance of organic syndromes.

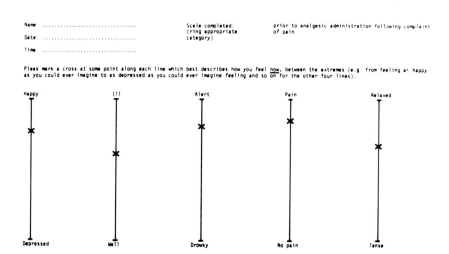

Figure 1 An analogue scale assessment which measures the emotional components of pain and the relationship between the degree of pain and degree of emotion

CRANIO-FACIAL PAIN

Psychological factors are particularly common in facial pain. Gerschman *et al.*[5] reported obvious psychiatric illness in the majority of 250 patients presenting with orofacial pain. Eighty per cent were treated with psychotherapy and 50% by drug therapy. Hypnotherapy was used in 26% and by these and other treatments they claimed a 70% 'marked alleviation' of symptoms in these patients. It is remarkable however that in this large series of patients no mention is made of surgical treatment and one must conclude that organic disorders such as symptomatic and idiopathic trigeminal neuralgia did not occur.

Trigeminal neuralgia is usually unilateral, affecting the maxillary or mandibular divisions in 70%. When Frazier[6] refined retrogasserian ganglionectomy this successful procedure became a standard neurosurgical operation, successfully relieving pain in the vast majority (re-operation was required in 7.5%), with a relatively low mortality although the deep anaesthesia produced was unpleasant to many, and facial dysaesthesiae occurred in about 14%. There were other admittedly small risks from craniotomy and since the operation was commonly performed in the elderly and often in the sitting position, hypotensive episodes in surgery were not uncommon. After the introduction of diphenylhydantoin and subsequently carbamazepine the number of trigeminal nerve sections performed fell in neurosurgical clinics throughout the world. These drugs successfully relieve trigeminal pain and can be prescribed until more definitive procedures are used. Drug idiosyncrasy and toxicity with giddiness and rashes however are common and increasing numbers of patients appear with pain recurrence despite adequate therapeutic blood levels. Control of the sharp lancinating pains is often effective although a deep aching pain may remain and induce the patient to increase his medication to toxic levels.

Alcoholic and phenolic injection of the ganglion is simple and safe and can be performed as an outpatient procedure but the alcohol produces profound anaesthesia and the risk of corneal anaesthesia is high whilst phenol is only a little less toxic.

A general desire to produce pain relief without accompanying anaesthesia encouraged the introduction of Dandy's[7] posterior fossa rhizotomy with section of the portio major which was believed to convey largely thermoalgesic sensation[8]. There is still controversy about whether pain fibres can be distinguished from others in the root and recent studies have indicated that such an arrangement is unlikely or at least not predominant. However, one possible advantage of a posterior fossa exposure is the revelation of tumours and vascular lesions. A microsurgical posterior fossa approach to the trigeminal nerve has been advocated by Jannetta[9]. He lists various causes for trigeminal neuralgia including herpes, sagging of the hind brain and demineralization of the skull base with angulation of the nerve root but finally concludes that pulsation of an arteriosclerotic carotid artery upon the nerve is the most likely cause of the tic douloureux. In his series of 100 patients he found compression by vascular structures in 88% and only 6% had compression by tumour or arteriovenous malformation. This high incidence of positive findings (94%) is held by some to indicate a readiness to accept as abnormalities appearances which may in fact be well within the normal range. Jennetta's present approach is that if he is unable to decompress the root by vascular mobilization then a selective nerve section is performed. Apfelbaum[10] has compared the treatment of 48 patients by percutaneous radiofrequency trigeminal rhizotomy with 55 patients treated by microvascular decompression via a posterior fossa exposure. In his series, 88% of patients with radiofrequency rhizotomy had successful initial relief of pain compared to 96% of patients with microvascular decompression. He also noted severe recurrence in 13% of patients with percutaneous rhizotomy and only 5% of those with microvascular decompression. In his series of percutaneous rhizotomies, however, his complication rate was higher than those reported by others. The fact that 15% of patients after microvascular decompression will require a second procedure compared to the situation with percutaneous rhizotomy where even if recurrence occurs it can be treated by an extremely simple and safe procedure, implies that for the majority of patients, radiofrequency rhizotomy is still the method of choice. For the young patient such an approach can be justified but since less than 1% of patients with trigeminal neuralgia are aged between 16 and 29 and only 9% are under 40, the indications are small[11].

Sweet and Wepsic[12] and Schurmann *et al.*[13] developed partial thermocoagulation of the trigeminal ganglion using the anterior approach of Hartel. This method, *radiofrequency rhizotomy*, has supplanted almost all other treatments of trigeminal neuralgia because of its efficacy, simplicity and safety. The patient is given a short-acting anaesthetic and the insulated electrode is introduced 3 cm lateral to the corner of the mouth with its tip directed to the intersection of a plane 3 cm anterior to the auditory meatus with that passing through the pupil (Figures 2 and 3). As the needle electrode enters the foramen ovale there is often a masseteric

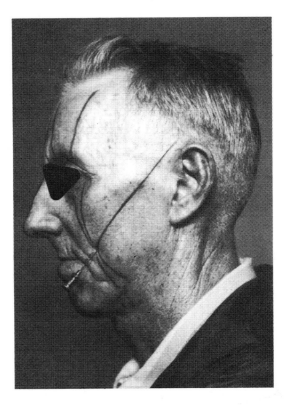

Figure 2 For percutaneous trigeminal rhizotomy the needle is introduced along a plane from 2.5 to 3 cm from the angle of the mouth to the midpoint of the zygoma and to the midpoint of the pupil

contraction and unilateral lachrymation. In more than 50% of patients it is possible to aspirate cerebrospinal fluid when the electrode stylet is removed. The position of the electrode can be confirmed by lateral and submento vertex radiographs but the response to electrical stimulation is much more reliable. Stimulation (0.2–0.5 V) at low frequencies (5 Hz) produces masseteric contraction whilst higher frequencies (50 Hz) produce tingling sensations in one, two or sometimes three divisions. According to the localization of these sensations the electrode is then adjusted to the depth at which stimulation produces response in the desired division and a radiofrequency lesion is made. This is best done by making an initial lesion of 60 °C for 60 seconds during which vasodilation of the face in one of the trigeminal divisions is common and confirms the correct siting of the electrode. If dense hypalgesia is not produced then the

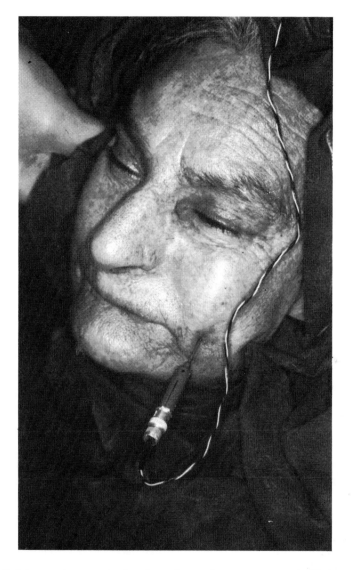

Figure 3 A temperature-monitoring electrode permits accurate control of lesion making

lesion is repeated at 5 °C higher or the electrode re-adjusted until a satisfactory sensory loss is obtained.

One particular advantage of the technique is that touch sensation is preserved or there is only a minimal loss compared to the analgesia produced[14]. This is particularly important when first division lesions are

141

produced since corneal anaesthesia is avoided and the corneal reflex is generally preserved. Siegfried[15] reported recurrence of only 4.3% in 500 patients during a follow-up period of one to 37 months and subsequently reported larger series with equally good results. There seems to be a greater chance of recurrence if analgesia is slight[16] and Sweet and Wepsic[12] found that 7% of their patients with inadequate sensory loss after the first procedure developed full pain recurrence and required further procedures. Touch sensation is preserved in over 80% of patients[17] which may be important in preventing postoperative dysaesthesia. Previous surgery is not a contraindication to this procedure although confirmation of puncture by CSF aspiration is less frequent if retrogasserian section has been performed.

Ericksson and Sjölund[18] suggest transcutaneous stimulation as an alternative treatment in chronic facial pain including trigeminal neuralgia. In 8 months follow up they reported 60% of patients obtained good pain relief. Siegfried and Haas[19] studying the effects of transcutaneous stimulation upon pain induced by heat stimulation in the trigeminal ganglion found that the pain threshold was increased. In practice, transcutaneous stimulation has a low rate of success and the facial electrodes are inconvenient and unsightly.

Peripheral radiofrequency neurectomy has also been introduced but has little, if any, advantages over rhizotomy and chances of re-innervation and pain recurrence appear to be greater. Cryoanalgesia using a fine cryoprobe has been advocated for a variety of intractable facial pains. Barnard *et al.*[20] used a fine cryoprobe in nine patients with post-herpetic neuralgia after exposing the nerve by dissection under local anaesthesia. The nerves were subsequently divided and the only advantage claimed for the method was that it permitted painless manipulation of nerves. In a second group of patients with atypical facial neuralgia, tic douloureux or malignant neuralgia, the nerves were frozen but not sectioned. In this latter group the median duration of pain relief was 116 days but the results are certainly no better than those for radiofrequency trigeminal rhizotomy.

Central lesions of the trigeminal pathway may also be useful. Kunc[21] has pointed out that the trigger zone of most patients with trigeminal neuralgia is in the central part of the face and fibres from this region terminate in the upper pole of the caudal nucleus of the trigeminal nerve. He interrupts the first and also the second order neurone by making a vertical incision along the medial margin of the trigeminal tract into the hilum of the caudal nucleus and is able to confine analgesia to the central portion of the face. Seventy-five per cent of his patients had a satisfactory result.

Percutaneous stereotactic trigeminal *tractotomy* and *nucleotomy* was introduced in 1968[22] as a method of producing widespread facial analgesia which can be extended into the greater part of the neck[23] (Figure 4). A fine electrode is introduced posteriorly over the arch of the atlas into the trigeminal tract and descending nucleus of the trigeminal nerve (Figure 5). Stimulation produces a sensory facial response and the nucleus is then destroyed by radiofrequency current. Schvarez[24] has reported 104 stereotactic nucleotomies and comments on its accuracy and safety. He advocates this for certain facial central pain phenomena including anaesthesia dolorosa. Fox[25] introduced a simple free-hand percutaneous trigeminal tractotomy and has reported good results. The small target and the dangers of injuring nearby structures however suggest that the stereotactic procedure is still one of choice.

Painful convulsive tic is a condition of hemifacial spasm and ipsilateral facial pain. It is usually associated with an ectatic vertebrobasilar arterial segment or less frequently with an arteriovenous malformation or cholesteatoma compressing the trigeminal and facial nerves in the posterior fossa[26]. Posterior fossa exploration and separation of the vascular anomaly from the nerve by microdissection may relieve this distressing syndrome and is a more rational approach to treatment than section of the trigeminal nerve or crushing of the facial nerve.

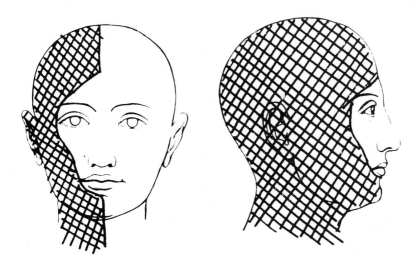

Figure 4 Typical area of analgesia produced by stereotactic trigeminal tractotomy and nucleotomy

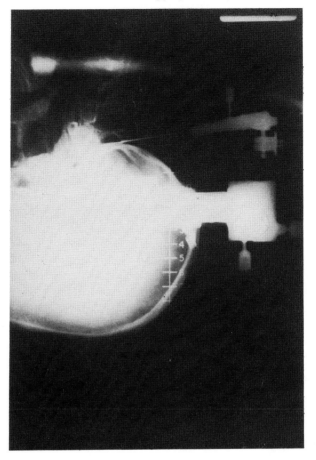

Figure 5 Introduction of a fine electrode into the cervical cord over the arch of the atlas

Glossopharyngeal and vagal neuralgias are typically tic-like but very difficult to evaluate. Swallowing or sneezing sets off the attack and the pain is at the back of the tongue, tonsillar fossa or posterior pharyngeal wall and often referred to the ear. The conditions are simply variants of disorders that can affect the trigeminal nucleus with activity in the upper portion of the nucleus producing classical tic douloureux and discharges in the lower portion producing pain in the ear or throat depending upon the part of the nucleus affected. There is considerable overlap between the lower afferent cranial nerves particularly and it is therefore often difficult to distinguish between glossopharyngeal and vagal neuralgia. The preferred method of treatment is complete section of the glosso-

144

pharyngeal nerve and the upper three vagal roots whilst Kunc[27] believes that bulbar tractotomy (trigeminal tractotomy) is the correct treatment. Both Tew[28] and Lazorthes and Verdie[29] have reported good results using a percutaneous radiofrequency method to destroy the ganglion. Swallowing difficulties are common after this procedure however and the method should probably be reserved for patients with secondary glossopharyngeal neuralgia from neoplasia. Laha and Jannetta[30] however have demonstrated vascular compression of the nerve by a tortuous vertebral or posterior inferior cerebellar artery and in selected patients microvascular decompression without nerve section can be curative.

Nervus intermedius neuralgia is characterized by brief tic-like attacks of pain within the ear and longer attacks which may go on for several hours. The treatment of choice is microsurgical exposure of the nerve via the posterior fossa. Identification of the nerve is not always easy and indeed ear pain may be due to diseases of other nerves such as the glossopharyngeal or vagus. Stimulation of the nerve with the patient aroused after a general anaesthetic for the exposure is valuable in identifying the nerve which produces the pain. In view of the numerous reports of vascular compression of these nerves the correct approach seems to be posterior fossa microsurgical exposure of the nerves to determine whether vascular or tumour compressions are the cause. If these are not found then section of the nerves should be done, preferably after stimulation studies have reproduced the patient's pain.

Meyerson and Haakansson[31] obtained good pain relief with transcutaneous nerve stimulation in 14 out of 25 patients with facial pain following trigeminal nerve section for tic douloureux, chronic sinusitis or post-operative dental pain. They therefore developed a method of direct stimulation of the Gasserian ganglion by placing a bipolar extradural electrode over it connected to a subcutaneous receiver. Five patients with atypical neuralgia from various causes experienced satisfactory pain relief over a follow up of between 6 months and 2 years.

The poor results reported from surgery for atypical facial pain have tended to detract attention from the fact that the term is often used to indicate facial pain which is not trigeminal neuralgia. In practice many facial pains may be revealed with distinct syndromes by careful history and examination. Although often searched for, tumours of the cerebellopontine angle do not usually produce facial pain but paranasal and posterior pharyngeal tumours commonly do. A radiofrequency rhizotomy offers a simple and often effective treatment for these disorders. Temporomandib-

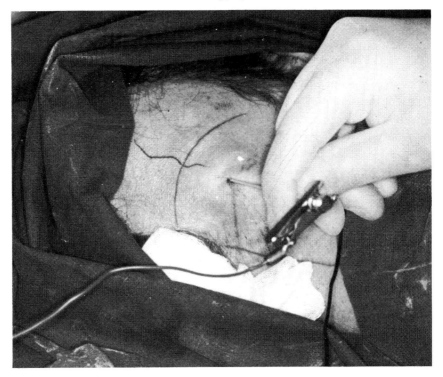

Figure 6 The needle is introduced 2 cm lateral to the midline at the bottom of the photograph, and 3 cm below the line of the occipital protruberance (semi-circular line). The course of the occipital nerve is marked by a wavy line

ular joint derangement may produce diffuse facial pain and can be diagnosed by demonstration of excessive movement of the condyle. Dental treatment by resetting the bite may produce relief but is not always effective and if symptoms are severe radiofrequency trigeminal rhizotomy should be offered. Autonomic faciocephalgia, a condition characterized by diffuse upper facial pain and associated lachrymation and facial flushing usually responds to ergotamine but intractable cases can be treated by petrosal nerve section via a temporal approach.

There is increasing recognition of the role of cervical spine disorder in producing referred facial pain which does not conform to the many syndromes now recognized. Cervical spondylosis should be considered as a possible cause. The association between facial pain and neck movements is rarely obvious but in a patient with facial pain associated with neck or shoulder pain, cervical nerve block should be attempted. If this produces relief, radiofrequency cervical facet neurectomy is worth a trial.

146

Occipital neuralgia is a condition of posterior head pain often due to so-called whip-lash injury. It may be suspected if there is a patchy sensory loss over the second cervical dermatome on one side and if pain is produced by vertex compression when the head is turned to the painful side. In the past this condition was treated by occipital nerve avulsion although posterior C_2 and C_3 rhizotomy is more successful. Blume[32] has introduced a simple percutaneous procedure using a radiofrequency current which can be performed as an outpatient procedure. In 250 patients with a follow-up from one to 4 years 75% had excellent results with complete abolition of pain and 5% had good results. An insulated needle is inserted 2 cm lateral to, and 3 cm below the occipital protuberance on the affected side and advanced cranially at a 45° angle to the skin until the tip touches the bone. Stimulation produces a tingling in the area and a radiofrequency lesion (85° for 120 seconds) is made (Figure 6).

TRUNK AND PELVIC PAIN

Back pain is a common symptom in general practice and a common cause of referral to specialist orthopaedic, neurosurgical and pain relieving clinics. There is little doubt that the vast majority of patients with acute prolapsed lumbar intervertebral discs respond well to strict bed rest with calf muscle exercise. If pain and disability are unrelieved, however, then laminectomy (usually through a small fenestration) and removal of the prolapsed fragment is required, the result of such surgery being excellent. Shannon[33] reviewed 325 patients with lumbar discs operated upon over a 10 year period. All patients had failed to respond to non-operative treatment and all had myelographic evidence of protrusion. Only 15 had recurrence at the previously operated level and were re-operated on after myelographic evidence of protrusion. Only 6 of these still have pain which is relieved by mild analgesics and after a 4 year follow-up all were still working.

The apparent high incidence of post-laminectomy pain is not substantiated by recent reports[34]. A relatively common problem is the patient presenting with backache with or without sciatica and where myelography reveals lumbar adhesions and arachnoiditis. The results of re-exploration and freeing of adhesions have not encouraged the widespread use of these techniques for these patients but Wilkinson and Schuman[35] reporting on 17 patients who had surgical lysis for lumbar adhesions and arachnoiditis noted improvement in pain in 76% and good to excellent relief in 35%. Although these figures fell to 50% still with some pain relief and only 25% with good to excellent pain relief, relief persisted in four out of five patients followed up for more than five years. This careful survey suggests that the generally dismal attitude to the treatment of lumbar arachnoiditis should be replaced with a more energetic approach although clearly the incidence of success will not be high and careful patient selection is of great importance. Law *et al.*[36] found that re-operation after failure of lumbar disc surgery produced successful pain relief in only 28% of patients but they noted that patients who had sensory loss involving more than one dermatone or who had no myelographic dural sac indentation did poorly after re-operation as did patients with past or pending compensation claims. However, if a herniated disc was found at re-operation the success rate was approximately 37%. These papers suggest that before resorting to analgesic surgery, exploration of the lumbar spine should be seriously considered and in cases where no disc protrusion is found it seems reasonable to perform a posterior rhizotomy of the affected roots. The chances of success however are not high. Onofrio and Campa[37] obtained only 13% success in such cases after posterior rhizotomy. Undoubtedly some back pain is associated with the degenerative changes which take place in the facetal joints which are often secondary to changes in the intervertebral disc. Rees[38] divided the nerve to the facet and claimed impressive results. Subsequently radiofrequency denervation was introduced[39] which was a more convenient method of destroying the nerve. Recently however there has been doubt cast as to whether such lesions made either with knife or radiofrequency have in fact denervated the target nerve. The most reliable method[40] is to direct the electrodes to the dorsal surface of the root of the transverse process immediately below the most medial end of its superior edge since here the nerve lies within 5 mm of the electrode tip. Having inserted the electrode, antero-posterior and lateral X-rays are taken and the nerve is stimulated. The method is very simple and safe and Shealy[39] quotes 79% of relief in patients without previous operations and 41% in patients after laminectomy.

Percutaneous posterior rhizotomy is difficult to perform in these cases because of the distortion of roots from the previous operation but is a relatively straightforward procedure[41, 42]. With the patient in position with the affected side uppermost a needle is introduced 4–5 cm from the midline and advanced towards the intervertebral foramen (Figure 7). Although it is helpful to do this under image intensification in my experience it is rarely necessary. It is usually possible to aspirate

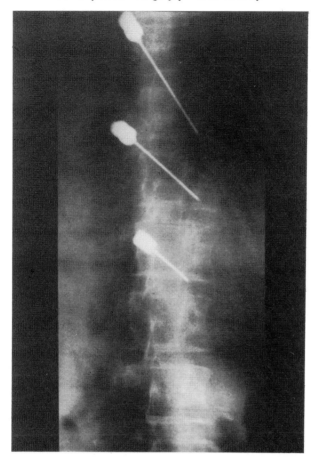

Figure 7 Percutaneous posterior rhizotomy. Needle advanced towards intervertebral foramen

cerebrospinal fluid which helps to confirm electrode position and the needle is then retracted until CSF can no longer be aspirated and electrical stimulation applied. The patient experiences tingling in the distribution of the nerve root and a radiofrequency lesion made. Such lesions commonly produce little or no sensory loss having the same effect as radiofrequency lesions in the trigeminal ganglion with the larger myelinated fibres relatively well preserved.

Pain in patients with carcinoma of the breast is generally due either to local invasion of the chest wall, axilla or supraclavicular region due to metastatic bone disease at various sites. Treatment of local disease is

149

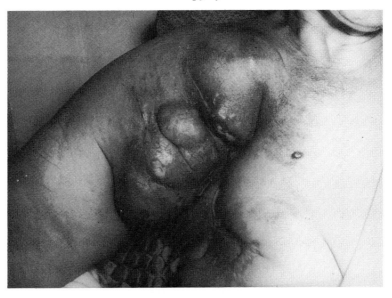

Figure 8 The appearances of gross invasive disease contributes to the general distress caused by pain. This patient complained of severe pain but detailed enquiry revealed her distress was more due to the massive swelling and odour of an invasive breast cancer

often complicated by infection and the visible evidence of gross recurrence which is often extremely disturbing to the patient (Figure 8). These emotional consequences must be considered in every case and dealt with by simple psychotherapy or the use of psychotropic drugs or else other methods used to control pain will be ineffective. Adequate analgesia of the affected areas can only be produced by extensive posterior rhizotomy since the surgeon must anticipate further extension and plan to include areas not presently affected. Because of the extensive overlap of innervation an adequate rhizotomy must include roots from C_4 to T_4[43]. The resulting sensory denervation of the arm produces a marked functional disability although some compensation occurs by visual aiding. Involvement of lower thoracic dermatomes is also common so that only denervation to T_8 is likely to be effective in most cases.

A number of studies[44] have shown that small and large fibres separate before entering the cord so that the nociceptor fibres run on the lateral side of the posterior root and the myelinated fibres run medially. Using this concept the procedure of selective *posterior rhizotomy* has been developed[45]. After an open exposure of the posterior roots an incision is made beneath the retracted posterior root, between root and cord about

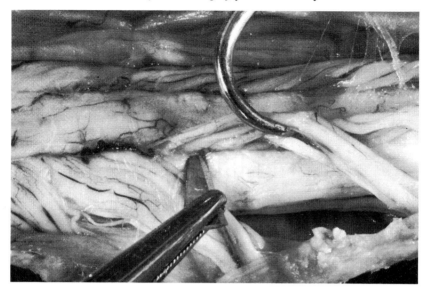

Figure 9 The posterior roots are retracted and a 2–3 mm deep incision made below their entry into the cord

2 mm deep (See Figure 9). By this selective technique it is claimed that only analgesia is produced and that the preservation of large fibre sensation tends to inhibit pain whilst the preservation of ordinary sensation preserves function of the extremities. Percutaneous radiofrequency posterior rhizotomy however also tends to produce a predominantly nociceptive loss and ordinary sensation is frequently preserved. In the case of posterior denervation for carcinoma of the breast the patient is placed on the side with the affected side uppermost and an insulated electrode is introduced through a spinal needle into the intervertebral foramina at thoracic and lower cervical dermatomes. This extensive rhizotomy is rather difficult technically and it may be necessary to repeat the procedure. For wide areas of involvement therefore other measures may be preferable.

Although pain due to metastatic tumours may be treated by appropriate denervation the areas are usually multiple and widely separated so that this approach is difficult. Certain breast and prostatic tumours however are at least partially hormone dependent and may respond to endocrine therapy. It is however interesting that in many patients who do not have hormone dependent tumours, hypophysectomy is still capable of producing pain relief[46].

If tumour regression as well as pain relief is to be attempted then microsurgical trans-sphenoidal hypophysectomy is indicated but in other cases, particularly those with metastatic disease and pain from other tumours, a simpler percutaneous approach may be sufficient. A percutaneous technique introduced by Forest *et al.*[47] for the insertion of radioactive yttrium has been used by Moricca[48] to destroy the gland by the injection of alcohol. Although he suggests that standard methods of hypophysectomy for carcinoma of the breast require costly apparatus and highly specialized staff the method advocated is unlikely to be used other than by specialized staff and is not without danger. The success of this method in producing pain relief in a wide variety of neoplasms is attributed to pituitary stalk destruction as compared to other methods which are generally limited to removal of, or destruction of the gland alone. Others[49,50] also record good results but Martino and Ventafridda[51] comparing the results of Moricca's methods with intramuscular high dose progesterone found that the latter was more effective in reducing pain in their study of 84 patients. They also noted arrest of carcinoma of the breast in 30% of their patients compared to pituitary neurolysis where no arrest was demonstrated.

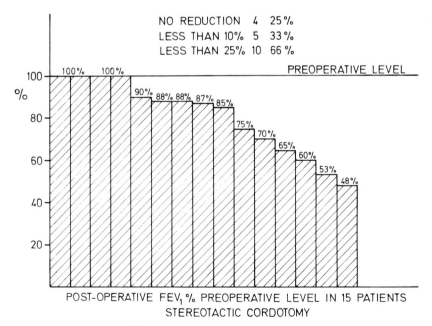

Figure 10 Stereotactic cordotomy

Pain due to carcinoma of the bronchus is felt in the chest due to direct invasion of the pleura or in the shoulder or arm due to invasion of the brachial plexus by tumour or malignant nodes. Open or percutaneous posterior rhizotomy effectively deals with thoracic and cervical dermatome pain but the commonly wide involvement encourages the use of a single procedure if possible. The particular complication of cordotomy, which must be a high cervical procedure in order to achieve high levels of analgesia, is that of respiratory disorder following surgery. The descending respiratory fibres have been shown[52] to pass close to and in part mixed with spinothalmic fibres from the trunk and arm. In conventional open cordotomy these fibres are invariably severed with the result that innervation of the relatively normal side is destroyed. The combination of mechanical respiratory dysfunction on one side and neuronal injury on the other produces gross disorders of pulmonary function. Although these can be avoided by a relatively superficial open cordotomy, percutaneous methods, particularly stereotactic cordotomy, are very much safer. Even with the small, accurate lesions produced by the stereotactic technique, cordotomy in patients with pre-existing respiratory disease is risky and if the FEV is less than 1.2 litres other methods such as

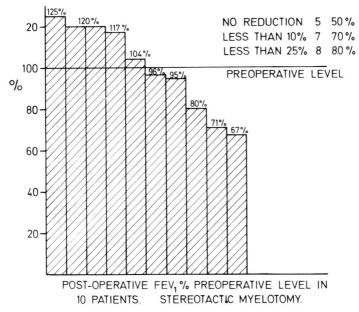

Figure 11 Stereotactic myelotomy

153

rhizotomy, myelotomy or thalamotomy should be considered (Figures 10 and 11). Lin *et al.*[53] introduced anterior low cervical percutaneous cordotomy to avoid injury to the respiratory pathways but the procedure is not popular because readjustments of electrode position are technically difficult and high analgesic levels cannot be obtained.

Intercostal neuralgia occurs in elderly patients with osteophytic compression of thoracic nerve roots and in others it is commonly due to injury to the nerve during thoracotomy. It is important to establish that the pain is a true neuralgia and not due to pain in other structures such as muscle in which case an extensive rhizotomy is required to produce analgesia, with section of two roots above and two roots below the affected dermatome or myotome in addition to section of the affected root. If percutaneous rhizotomy produces only transient relief then open rhizotomy should be considered and with pain of unequivocal single root distribution a single rhizotomy should suffice. *Post-herpetic truncal neuralgia* is another common syndrome and if it persists longer than a few months after the erruption surgery should be considered. The diagnosis is readily made from the history and from finding the characteristic scars in the affected dermatomes. On careful enquiry patients will often reveal that the pain has two distinct components; a superficial burning pain associated with extreme surface tenderness and a more diffuse deep aching pain. Superficial hyperpathia can be abolished by posterior rhizotomy but the deep pain often remains and may be more intense. Occasionally a radiofrequency lesion in the substantia gelatinosa will relieve this pain permanently but many patients are satisfied with relief of the superficial pain and hyperpathia, particularly if warned that some deep pain may remain if only a peripheral procedure is done. In my experience a combination of posterior rhizotomy which relieves the hyperpathia and superficial pain and chlorpromazine or some other psychotropic drug provides effective relief for the vast majority.

Abdominal pain from visceral disease or abdominal scars is often very difficult to deal with. One of the major problems is making an accurate diagnosis. Before any analgesic surgery is contemplated the diagnosis should be very carefully reviewed and any investigations which have been omitted should be performed. Pain due to involvement of intercostal nerves responds well to posterior rhizotomy[45] either percutaneous or by open surgery. Abdominal pain due to cancer is often a complex presentation of visceral pain and somatic pain. When disease is limited to the organ then sympathectomy gives transient relief but invasion of the posterior abdominal wall usually soon occurs with pain recurrence. A combination of coeliac plexus block and posterior rhizotomy however may deal with these situations. Posterior rhizotomy is usually successful for the relief of abdominal pain due to operation scars provided it is sufficiently extensive but because of the extensive denervation required percutaneous rhizotomy should be attempted first.

Coccydynia can be an incapacitating and puzzling complaint which is rarely relieved by resection of the coccyx which, indeed, commonly enhances the pain. Bilateral fourth and fifth sacral and coccygeal rhizotomy may relieve this pain without producing anal incontinence but psychological disorders are common in this condition and very careful patient selection is necessary. Presacral neurectomy and other pelvic denervations are now rarely indicated for dysmenorrhoea which usually responds well to hormonal treatment.

The problems of *pelvic and perineal pain* demand special care and attention and this is one of the most difficult areas to treat. Carcinoma of the cervix, prostate and rectum produce visceral pain which is often diffuse and poorly localized and is transmitted via the parasympathetic inflow of S_2 to S_5. When the disease extends into the adjacent lumbosacral plexus a more defined and often midline perineal or leg pain is produced. Well-localized pain can be treated by third, fourth and fifth sacral and coccygeal rhizotomies or by cordotomy, although in both cases there is a considerable risk of producing urinary retention or incontinence. In practice this latter is not always a contraindication to the procedure since so many of these patients already have serious urinary difficulties and the complication can often be ignored because the patient is either catheterized or is likely to require catheterization because of spread of the disease. The risk of urinary disorder however is particularly high when the pain is perineal and when bilateral involvement has occurred. Crue and Todd[54] have described a simple sacral rhizotomy at the first piece of the sacrum with extradural ligation and section of the dural sheath below the emergence of the S_4 root. The method is not recommended however if there is any leg pain and if bladder function is to be retained then the second sacral root must be preserved. Despite these precautions bladder function is almost invariably affected. If bilateral rhizotomy is attempted and both S_2 and S_3 roots are damaged then urinary and rectal incontinence will occur and although many cases have colostomy and catheter the risk of producing rectal incontinence particularly, is one that may make this method unacceptable for certain cases. This risk is considerably less with cordotomy and the lower complication rate for stereotactic and percutaneous procedures make these the methods of choice.

155

Because the pain is so commonly bilateral, attempts have been made to divide the decusating fibres of the spinothalamic tract. This procedure *myelotomy* was introduced by Armour in 1927 at the cervical level but it became established as an open thoracolumbar incision and is often performed for abdominopelvic or perineal pain. The advantages of myelotomy are the lower incidence of urinary retention and leg weakness because injury to the descending micturition fibres and corticospinal pathways is less likely. The incision must be made at least three segments higher than the highest affected dermatome because spinothalamic fibres require one to three segments to cross the cord. The incision is usually two to four centimetres long and Sourek[55] who performed thoracic myelotomy in 36 patients reported complete relief in 31 although all had transient urinary difficulties. Only four patients were unrelieved and in those the pain was then higher and of a different quality. The advantages of this method for bilateral pain and for patients with sphincter disturbances is obvious. The analgesia produced varies from case to case but Sourek found that anogenital pain could be relieved by thoracic myelotomy. He also noted that spontaneous pain was relieved even in areas with normal pin prick sensation, which he attributed to injury of the medial parts of the dorsal columns. Lembcke[56] re-introduced cervical myelotomy for 12 patients with arm and leg pain and in 1970[57] *stereotactic cervical myelotomy* was introduced. These single lesions produced at the first cervical segment resulted in pain relief and analgesia which included the lower half of the body (Figure 12). This widespread alteration of pain sensitivity suggested that the interruption was not only of decusating spinothalamic fibres but also of a multi-synaptic central system conveying slower conducting pain sensation. Grade 1 (no pain, no analgesics) pain relief[58], was achieved in 90% at hospital discharge which fell to 64% relieved at 3 months. Thereafter survivors maintained grade 1 or grade 2 (infrequent pain, complete relief by weak, non-narcotic analgesics) until death or last follow-up which in one case was for more than 5 years. Schvarez[59] noted excellent relief in 45 patients following this procedure. Although transient ataxia is common there is no mortality and a low (less than 1%) incidence of bladder dysfunction. King[60] estimated that 60 to 70% of patients are relieved of bilateral lower half and midline pain whilst sphincter disturbances, monoparesis and paraparesis are rare. Cook and Kawakami[61] however concluded that the procedure had outstanding advantages for patients with bilateral malignancies but was less effective for those with intrapelvic malignancy.

Open lumbosacral myelotomy and stereotactic cervical myelotomy are

156

performed more frequently and recently Eiras *et al.*[62] have used a simple percutaneous aiming technique to perform cervical myelotomy in 12 patients with malignant pain. From their observations they conclude that the effect was the same as that obtained by stereotatic lesions of the centremedian complex. Schvarez[24] has performed cervical myelotomy on 75 patients and achieved satisfactory pain relief in 78% of patients with pain due to neoplasia which confirms my own experience[58]. Myelotomy either by the stereotactic cervical procedure or the open lumbosacral operation provides a useful new method of dealing with bilateral pain, particularly that due to pelvic malignancy.

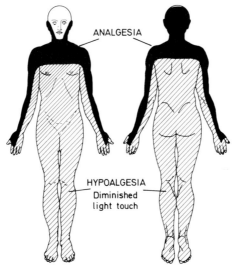

03.07.92. J.R. Open C1/2 RF Myelotomy 1-6-72
Sensory findings 19-6-72

Figure 12 Profound and extensive analgesia produced by a single C1/2 central cord lesion

EXTREMITY PAIN

Arm or leg pain due to tumour, fractures, nerve injury or soft tissue trauma and from accident or surgery requires a careful search for the exact site of pain and differentiation between nerve or other tissue involved. The large overlap of innervation implies extensive denervation for pain in addition to that due to specific nerve root involvement. Peripheral neurectomy is sometimes successful but a limited posterior rhizotomy is probably better. It is wise to perform an anaesthetic block prior to resection to determine individual variation of innervations to deep and superficial structures, but Sindou *et al.*[45] quote relief of 50% in 20 patients reported in the literature. The concern with posterior rhizotomy in the arm is the risk of sensory paresis and if complete dysfunction is to be avoided then C_6 or C_7 or both C_5 and C_8 must be kept intact. These restrictions impose considerable drawbacks in the management of most patients with arm pain since it so commonly involves more than two dermatomes. In the case of lower limb pain L_2, L_3 or L_4 must be preserved to retain quadriceps stability. Percutaneous rhizotomy is a procedure of choice for malignant pain since although there is a higher rate of recurrence, most patients will have died before this becomes a problem.

In the past the treatment for pain in the flail anaesthetic limb produced by brachial plexus avulsion was amputation but this crude procedure is almost invariably unsuccessful. Although pain is common following brachial plexus avulsion and occurs within 48 hours of injury it usually gradually disappears. Zorab *et al.*[63] reviewing 50 patients with brachial plexus avulsion found that 20% had intractable pain whilst for patients with total plexus lesions this incidence increased to 67%. Cervical lissauer tractotomy and gelatinosa nucleotomy[58] has successfully relieved phantom arm pain following brachial plexus avulsion. The electrode is introduced with the aid of a simple electrode carrier fitted to muscle retractors used in the laminectomy exposure (Figure 13). Nashold and Ostdhal[64] have recently reported results with dorsal root entry zone lesions in 21 patients with arm pain due to plexus avulsion, in whom 13 (67%) had good pain relief over a period of 6 months to 3½ years. They believe that in patients with plexus avulsion, pain is produced from pathophysiological changes in the injured dorsal horn of the spinal cord explaining the failure of peripheral procedures such as rhizotomy and sympathectomy. Cordotomy or thalamotomy may be more suitable in some cases and Zorab *et al.*[63] had good results with mesencephalotomy. Dorsal column stimulation was generally ineffective however.

White and Sweet[65] reporting the response to a questionnaire and a review of the literature of more than 3000 percutaneous cordotomies compared with 355 personal cases of open cordotomy found that initially analgesia and pain relief were similar (82% and 81%). Thereafter however few percutaneous procedures were followed up for more than 6 months. After open cordotomy 70% were relieved of pain for 6 months and 50% for from 1 to 32 years. The mortality however was higher for open operations than for percutaneous and complications were more frequent. They concluded that percutaneous cordotomy was the correct

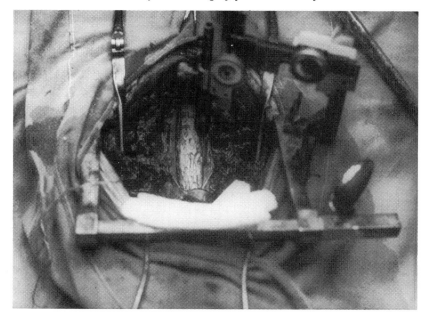

Figure 13 Simple electrode holder for root entry zone lesions

procedure for malignant pain but for those with pain from other causes open cordotomy was preferable. Open high cervical cordotomy is more suitable than the older thoracic cordotomy since complications are fewer and higher levels of analgesia can be produced.

Percutaneous aiming or stereotactic cordotomy is often the correct procedure for patients with malignancies. Tasker[66] reported 96% immediate pain relief falling to 85% at the time of the latest (undefined) follow-up after percutaneous cordotomy. For bilateral cordotomy relief was obtained in 68%. 19% of patients had transient paresis and 6% of the unilateral procedures and 21% of bilateral procedures had aggravated bladder dysfunction. Some of these complications may be reduced by using a stereotactic procedure to place the electrode with greater accuracy in the spinal cord. The procedure is more complex than the relatively straightforward percutaneous method but it is especially useful for patients where the risk of bladder or respiratory complications is particularly high. The results of stereotactic cordotomy are superior to the cruder percutaneous procedure[58] but the former requires special instrumentation and training. Both percutaneous and stereotactic cordotomy need a co-operative patient without confusion or emotional lability while cervical spine deformity, infection or tumours can make this procedure

159

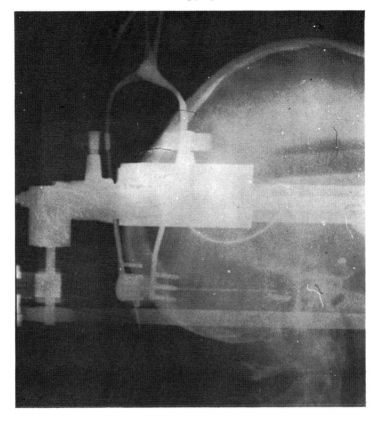

Figure 14 Lateral X-ray of electrode within spinothalamic tract at pontine level

quite unsuitable. For those reasons open cordotomy still offers a safe and effective method of pain relief when percutaneous procedures are unacceptable. Stereotactic pontine tractotomy[67] (Figure 14) is rarely necessary but is a useful procedure when high sensory levels are required and where the risk of respiratory or urinary disorder is particularly high. Cassinari and Pagni[2] have commented on the rarity of central pain and dysaesthesia following bulbo-spinothalamic tractotomy which they attributed to interruption of polysynaptic reticulospinal fibres along with the spinothalamic.

Although phantom limbs are common amongst amputees, happily phantom limb pain is relatively uncommon. The patient complains of pain usually in the distal portion of the amputated limb and often describes a painful abnormal posture of hand or foot. If spinal anaesthesia completely removes the pain then cordotomy may be suc-

160

cessful without however changing the shape or size of the phantom. Unfortunately pain tends to recur in some patients after a variable interval from months to years and in most cases unilateral thalamotomy should be considered. Dorsal column stimulation has been used frequently but the long term results are generally poor.

Peripheral nerve injuries are sometimes followed by severe burning pain characteristically exacerbated by stress or temperature change and termed causalgia by Weir Mitchell in 1864. The exact causation of this pain has been the subject of extensive investigation and discussion for many years but it is now accepted that the role of the sympathetic pathway in this condition is efferent rather afferent. Earlier theories suggested that artificial synapses permitted stimulation of somatic axons by efferent sympathetic fibres thus explaining the efficacy of sympathectomy. Recent studies suggest rather that increased amounts of noradrenaline are produced which act on sensitive nerves to produce pain. Sympathectomy, which is very effective in the treatment of causalgia, should always be preceded by a diagnostic block and White[68] states that the success rate should exceed 90% with good patient selection. Although operative sympathectomy is more accurate and long lasting it is reasonable to try chemical sympathectomy first. If causalgia is relieved but recurs after a reasonable interval then the open procedure can be approached with greater confidence.

Sympathectomy is also useful in the treatment of visceral disease provided somatic innervation is not involved. Thus it can effectively remove pain due to pancreatic disease although not if the posterior parietal peritoneum is involved; splanchnectomy must be bilateral for these patients. White[68] has pointed out the concentration of visceral afferent fibres in splanchnic trunks and paravertebral sympathetic ganglionic chains. Because grafting of coronary arteries is increasingly performed sympathectomy for heart pain is less common and obviously less preferable but where this is not possible then resection of the upper thoracic ganglia can be offered. The same remarks apply to sympathectomy for aortic aneurysm where alcoholic injection of the upper two thoracic ganglia can be performed but where direct surgical attack upon the aneurysm is more usual. Thoracic splanchnectomy may be done for pain due to adhesions following laparotomy and post-cholecystectomy neuralgia can be relieved by resection of the hepatic nerve plexus via the bed of the right eleventh rib. The same authors[69] suggest splanchnic resection of the upper lumbar chain via the bed of the twelfth rib to totally denervate the kidney and ureter for pain. Hupert[70] has pointed out the frequency with which cancer may produce causalgia and reported a group of cancer patients who were successfully relieved of pain by sympathetic denervation having previously been unresponsive to all forms of therapy.

CNS ELECTRICAL STIMULATION

I have chosen to discuss stimulation of the central nervous system separately since although many procedures have been performed and good results reported, recent papers have been less enthusiastic and the suggested mechanisms of action are controversial. At the present time opinion is divided as to whether the effect is due to blocking the pain pathways or more fashionably to the production of opiate-like substances. The prolonged effect of relatively brief stimulation seems to favour the latter view but recent reports have suggested that this might not be the case. Further experience and study is necessary before electrical stimulation of the CNS for pain relief can be established and before classical destructive methods can be entirely replaced. This is especially important when we consider the expense of these devices which at present is over one thousand pounds for each implantation and which are followed by a high incidence of mechanical defects.

Campbell and Long[71] implanted major nerves in the area of the patient's pain in 33 cases and reported dramatic success in patients with peripheral nerve injury. The most popular method of electrical stimulation, however, is spinal stimulation although the long term results have been disappointing[72]. Reviewing the results of dorsal column stimulation in 489 patients reported in the literature by 1975, Long[73] found only 18% with excellent relief of pain and 37% with satisfactory relief.

Stimulators were originally implanted by open laminectomy and placed on the dorsal column of the spinal cord but this has been supplanted by percutaneous epidural procedures which permit long-term evaluation of stimulation so that the final permanent implantation is only done in patients where stimulation has successfully relieved the pain over a period. Urban and Nashold[74] concluded that percutaneous epidural stimulation was a satisfactory alternative to dorsal column stimulation. Describing their experience in 70 patients[75] with pain due to multiple sclerosis and other chronic diseases they concluded that percutaneous epidural stimulation had no major complications and was a relatively simple procedure.

Black and North[76] found that 28% (five) of 18 patients obtained 'moderate to excellent' pain relief by spinal epidural electrical stimulation over an average follow up of 11 months but recurrence or replacement of the stimulating system was necessary in 6 out of the 18 (33%) because of mechanical failure. North and Long[77] recorded 64 minor surgical procedures necessary because of electrode migration, lead fracture and transmitter or antennae failure in 23 patients.

The implantation should be carried out in the operating room under local anaesthesia and using a sterile technique. Tuohy needles are inserted through the spinous interspaces into the epidural space identified by the negative pressure method. The flexible electrodes are then inserted through the needle until they lie with their tips one or two spaces above the needle tips. The position can be checked with X-ray but the patient's response to stimulation is the major guide. The electrodes are then manipulated until sensations are produced in the painful area and 24 hours later stimulation test programmes are begun. It is very important to ensure that the patient performs the very first stimulation since reliance on nursing or medical staff to adjust the stimulator produces considerable difficulties in later management. One of the major contraindications for the use of these complex methods is patient confusion or lack of intelligence which prevents even the simple manipulation of the stimulator which is required.

The results of brain stimulation for relief of pain is more controversial and more difficult to assess. Adams *et al.*[78] stimulated the posterior limb of the internal capsule in 30 patients with intractable pain and in three of them obtained continued pain relief after only 3 days stimulation. In 15 other patients the result of percutaneous stimulation was sufficiently encouraging to internalize the stimulating system and in 12 patients with central pain four were completely relieved and six obtained sufficient relief to continue stimulation. Mazars *et al.*[79] in an important paper presented their experience with 414 electrode stimulations and noted that analgesia was never produced with stimulation at non-blocking levels, and naloxone reversal was never convincing. Mazars now believes that analgesia produced by stimulation of the peri-aqueductal grey region is due to neuronal blocking of the spinothalamic tract. Cosyns[80] reporting his experience of peri-aqueductal and medial thalamic stimulation noted that after stimulation of 28 different electrode points only one patient had significant relief of pain and in others stimulation was ineffective. Such lack of success for stimulation has been criticized as being due to poor placement of the electrodes but Gybels *et al.*[81], similarly disappointed with the results of such stimulation, had an opportunity of checking electrode position after death which revealed that placement was correct. Others[82] have been more enthusiastic and Ray and Burton[83] reported 75% success in 25 patients. Hosobuchi[84] reported his experience of brain stimulation in 56 patients. Twenty of 39 patients with deafferentiation pain (thalamic syndrome, anaesthesia dolorosa, postherpetic neuralgia etc.) had satisfactory pain control by stimulation alone. Over 6 months to 8 years of follow-up 14 of these 20 patients had total relief by brain stimulation alone. These results were achieved with stimulation of the thalamus, posterior limb of the internal capsule and the medial lemniscus but in 17 of these patients a second electrode implanted into the peri-aqueductal grey matter failed to give any pain relief. In contrast, the 17 patients with pain due to peripheral disorders such as cancer or back pain obtained total relief by peri-aqueductal grey stimulation but seven patients were considered therapeutic failures within 2–20 months. Richardson and Akil[85] found that stimulation of the peri-aqueductal grey matter relieved pain but produced unpleasant side effects such as oculomotor disorders. Medial thalamic stimulation however had few unpleasant side effects and produced good pain relief. Review of the results of such procedures in more than 200 patients collected from various European clinics[86] showed that the outcome of treatment appeared to be highly unpredictable and at the present time the insertion of these devices which require stereotactic instrumentation and expertise will necessarily be limited to a few clinics where their use can be evaluated.

CEREBRAL TARGETS

At the present time the results of destruction of the areas which have been treated with stimulation to produce pain relief show consistently better results.

Stereotactic mesencephalotomy is a useful method of dealing with unilateral or bilateral pain due to carcinoma of the head, neck and arm areas[87] and has also been advocated for thalamic syndrome and phantom limb pain. The electrode is aimed at a target point 5 mm behind and below the posterior commisure and 5 to 10 mm from the midline. Unfortunately oculomotor defects and post-operative dysaesthesia are common complications and can be extremely troublesome.

Basal *thalamotomy* where the lesion is made a little higher has a somewhat lower incidence of complications and shows particularly good results in the relief of central pain. Centre-median thalamotomy destroys the medial posterior thalamic nuclear relay and is generally superior to basal thalamotomy, especially if bilateral procedures are performed whilst complications are less frequent.

The patient is placed in a sitting or semi-recumbent position on the operating table and the stereotactic instrument applied under local anaesthesia supplemented with small doses of intravenous Diazepam. The ventricles are outlined with a watermiscible dye and the thalamic target measured in respect to the AC–PC line and referred to the stereotactic grid. The radiofrequency electrode is then introduced towards this target. Stimulation at or near the target site frequently produces pain in the contralateral part of the body. This physiological confirmation of electrode position is often very useful. Stimulation of centremedian more commonly produces a generalized unpleasant sensation. Richardson and Akil[88] have suggested that the centremedian nucleus acts as a part of the gating mechanism transmitting noxious stimulae. This concept of a generalized rather than a localized role in pain sensation encourages the view that bilateral lesions will be superior to unilateral. Watkins[89] reported 22 patients with benign pain treated by thalamotomy of whom 18 benefited. Eleven patients, however, required bilateral thalamotomy and all but two patients required further thalamic lesions after initial relief, then remaining pain free for an average of 5 years. Rodriguez-Burgos *et al.*[90], however, reporting on 22 patients who had bilateral cryo-thalamotomy of CM–PF reported 10 of 16 patients with malignancy who were free of pain until death within one year and suggest the procedure should be reserved for patients with malignancy. Laitenen[91] has had better results with pulvinotomy[92-94]. Seventy per cent of 68 patients with malignant and non-malignant pain were relieved by lesions in centre-median and dorsomedialis[95].

The fashion for thalamic stimulation rather than destruction has produced hesitation in considering patients for thalamotomy. However, the expense and vulnerability of electrical stimulation systems at the present time is discouraging and limiting and thalamotomy should not be dismissed without careful consideration.

Pain is a complex sensation with a strong emotional association and there is a great deal of evidence that the limbic system is an important participant. Limbic lesions therefore influence pain experience although they exercise their effect by disturbance of personality which, although slight, can be demonstrated by psychological testing. For certain patients such as those in terminal states with great anguish and distress associated with pain, a limited leukotomy or limbic lobe lesion can relieve pain that cannot be relieved by drugs[96]. Kuroda *et al.*[97] performed anterior cingulumotomy in 29 patients with malignant pain and found that 75% had relief from bilateral lesions and sixty-six per cent were relieved from unilateral lesions. Bilateral lesions relieved 77% of nine patients with non-malignant pain.

CONCLUSION

Recent surgical interest has been with non-destructive procedures but the wide variety of procedures available means that an operation may be chosen which is suitable for any particular patient's needs. Although percutaneous methods have replaced many open techniques some such as rhizotomy are being refined and produce excellent results.

References

1 Keller, J. T. (1977). *The Anatomy of Central Pain Pathways in Pain Management.* (Baltimore: Williams and Wilkins)

2 Cassinari, V. and Pagni, C. A. (1969). *Central Pain: A Neurological Survey.* p. 55. (Cambridge & Harrow University Press)

3 Nathan, P. W. (1963). Results of anterolateral cordotomy for pain in cancer. *J. Neurol. Neurosurg. Psychiatr.,* **26,** 353

4 French, L. A., Shou, S. N. and Story, J. L. (1966). Cervical tractotomy: techniques and clinical usefulness. In Knighton, R. S. and Dumke, P. R. (eds.) *Pain.* (Boston: Little Brown & Co.)

5 Gerschman, J. A., Burrows, G. D. and Reade, P. C. (1979). Chronic oro-facial pain. In: Bonica J. J. *et al.* (eds.). *Advances in Pain Research and Therapy.* Vol. 3, pp. 317–323. (New York: Raven Press)

6 Frazier, C. H. (1928). Operation for the radical cure of trigeminal neuralgia. Analysis of five hunred cases. *Ann. Surg.,* **88,** 534

7 Dandy, W. E. (1929). Operation for cure of tic douloureux; partial section of the sensory root at the pons. *Arch. Surg.,* **18,** 687

8 Provost, J. and Hardy, J. (1970). Microchirurgie due trijumeau: anatomie functionelle. *Neurochirurgie,* **16,** 459

9 Jannetta, P. J. (1976). Microsurgical approach to the trigeminal nerve for tic douloureux. *Prog. Neurol. Surg.,* **7,** 180

10 Apfelbaum, R. I. (1977). A comparison of percutaneous-radiofrequency trigeminal neurolysis and microvascular decompression of the trigeminal nerve for the treatment of tic douloureux. *Neurosurgery,* **1,** 16

11 Henderson, W. R. (1967). Trigeminal neuralgia: the pain and its treatment. *Br. Med. J.,* **1,** 7

12 Sweet, W. H. and Wepsic, J. C. (1974). Controlled thermocoagulation of trigeminal ganglion and rootlets for differential destruction of pain fibres. Part 1. Trigeminal neuralgia. *J. Neurosurg.,* **39,** 143

13 Schurmann, M., Butz, M. and Brock, M. (1972). Temporal retrogasserian resection of trigeminal root versus controlled elective percutaneous electrocoagulation of the ganglion of Gasser in the treatment of trigeminal neuralgia. Report on a series of 531 cases. *Acta Neurochir.*, **26,** 33

14 Sweet, W. H. (1975). Pain. Mechanisms and treatment. In Tower, D. B. (ed.). *The Nervous System. Vol. 2. The Classical Neurosciences.* pp. 487–500. (New York: Raven Press)

15 Siegfried, J. (1977). 500 percutaneous thermocoagulation of the gasserian ganglion for trigeminal pain. *Surg. Neurol.*, **8,** 126

16 Nugent, G. R. and Berry, B. (1974). Trigeminal neuralgia treated by differential percutaneous radiofrequency coagulation of the gasserian ganglion. *J. Neurosurg.*, **40,** 517

17 Onofrio, B. M. (1975). Radiofrequency percutneous gasserian ganglion lesions. *J. Neurosurg.*, **42,** 132

18 Eriksson, M. B. E. and Sjöland, B. H. (1978). Pain relief from conventional versus acupuncture-like T.N.S. in patients with chronic facial pain. In *Pain Abstracts.* Vol. 1, p. 128. Second World Congress on Pain. (Seattle: Int. Assoc. Study of Pain)

19 Siegfried, J. and Haas, H. L. (1978). Inhibition by transcutaneous electrical stimulation of noxious heat elicited in human Gasserian ganglion. In *Pain Abstracts.* Vol. 1, p. 128. Second World Congress on Pain. (Seattle: Int. Assoc. Study Pain)

20 Barnard, J. D. W., Lloyd, J. W. and Glynn, C. J. (1978). Cryosurgery in the management of intractable facial pain. *Br. J. Oral Surg.*, **16,** 135

21 Kunc, Z. (1979). Vertical trigeminal partial nucleotomy. In Bonica, J. J. *et al.* (eds.): *Advances in Pain Research and Therapy.* Vol. 3, pp. 325–330 (New York: Raven Press)

22 Hitchcock, E. (1970). Stereotactic trigeminal tractotomy. *Ann. Clin. Res.*, **2,** 131

23 Crue, B. L., Todd, E. M. and Carregal, E. J. (1970). Percutaneous radiofrequency stereotactic trigeminal tractotomy. In *Pain and Suffering.* pp. 69–79. (Springfield: C. C. Thomas)

24 Schvarez, J. R. (1978). Spinal cord stereotactic techniques re trigeminal nucleotomy and extralemniscal myelotomy. *Appl. Neurophysiol.*, **41,** 99

25 Fox, J. L. (1978). Percutaneous trigeminal tractotomy for facial pain. *Acta Neurochir.*, **29,** 83

26 Pulsinelli, W. A. and Rottenberg, D. A. (1977). Painful tick convulsif. *J. Neurol. Neurosurg. Psychiatr.*, **40,** 192

27 Kunc, Z. (1965). Treatment of essential neuralgia of the 9th nerve by selective tractotomy. *J. Neurosurg.*, **23,** 494

28 Tew, J. M. (1977). Percutaneous rhizotomy in the treatment of intractable facial pain (trigeminal, glossopharyngeal and vagus nerves). In Schmidek, H. H. and Sweet, W. H. (eds.) *Current Techniques in Operative Neurosurgery.* pp. 409–426. (New York: Grune and Stratton)

29 Lazorthes, Y. and Verdie, J. C. (1979). Radiofrequency coagulation of the petrous ganglion in glossopharyngeal neuralgia. *Neurosurgery*, **4,** 512

30 Laha, R. K. and Jannetta, P. J. (1977). Glossopharyngeal neuralgia. *J. Neurosurg.*, **47,** 316

31 Meyerson, B. A. and Haakansson, S. (1980). Alleviation of facial pain by stimulation of the Gasserian ganglion via an implanted electrode. In Proceedings of the European Society for Stereotactic and Functional Neurosurgery. *Acta Neurochir.* (In press)

32 Blume, H. G. (1978). Radiofrequency denaturation in occipital pain: a new approach in 250 cases. *Pain Abstracts.* Vol. 1. p. 143. 2nd World Congress on Pain. (Seattle: Int. Assoc. Study of Pain)

33 Shannon, N. (1978). Lumbar disc re-operation. *J. Neurosurg.*, **49,** 157

34 Rothman, R. H. (1978). Criteria for disectomy in patients with low back pain. *Pain*

Abstracts. Vol. 1, p. 221. Second World Congress on Pain. p. 221. (Seattle: Int. Assoc. Study of Pain)

35 Wilkinson, H. A. and Schuman, N. (1979). Results of surgical lysis of lumbar adhesive arachnoiditis. *Neurosurgery,* **4,** 401

36 Law, J. D., Lehman, R. A. W. and Kirsch, W. M. (1978). Re-operation after lumbar intravertebral disc surgery. *J. Neurosurg.,* **48,** 259

37 Onofrio B. M. and Campa. H. K. (1972). Evaluation of rhizotomy. Review of 12 years experience. *J. Neurosurg.,* **36,** 751

38 Rees, W. E. S. (1971). Multiple bilateral subcutaneous rhizolysis of segmental nerves in the treatment of the intravertebral disc syndrome. *Ann. Gen. Pract.,* **26,** 126

39 Shealy, C. N. (1975). Percutaneous radiofrequency denervation of spinal facets. *J. Neurosurg.,* **43,** 448

40 Bogduk, N. (1978). The surgical anatomy of lumbar zygapophyseal joint denervation. *Pain Abstracts.* Vol. 1. 2nd World Congress on Pain. (Seattle: Int. Assoc. Study of Pain)

41 Uematsu, S., Udvarrhely, G. B., Benson, D. W. and Siebens, A. A. (1974). Percutaneous radiofrequency rhizotomy. *Surg. Neurol.,* **2,** 319

42 Lazorthes, Y., Verdie, J. C. and Lagarrigue, J. (1976). Thermocoagulation percutanée des nerfs rachidiens à visée analgésique. *Neurochirurgie,* **22,** 445

43 Ray, B. S. (1943). The management of intractable pain by posterior rhizotomy. *Res. Nerv. Ment. Dis.,* **23,** 391

44 Spivy, D. F. and Metcalf. J. S. (1959). Differential effect of the medial and lateral dorsal root sections upon subcortical evoked potentials. *J. Neurophysiol.,* **22,** 373

45 Sindou, M., Fischer, G. and Mansuy, L. (1977). Posterior spinal rhizotomy and selective posterior rhizidiotomy. In Krayenbühl, H., Maspes, P. E. and Sweet, W. H. (eds.) Progress in Neurological Surgery, Volume 7, Part 1 p. 201 (Berlin: S. Karger)

46 Tindall, G. T., Nixon, D. W., Christy, J. H. and Neill, J. D. (1977). Pain relief in metastatic cancer other than breast and prostate gland following transphenoidal hypophysectomy. *J. Neurosurg.,* **47,** 659

47 Forest, A. P. M., Roberts, M. M. and Stewart, H. J. (1974). Pituitary ablation by yttrium 90. *Acta Neurochir.,* **21,** 137

48 Morica, G. (1974). Chemical hypophysectomy for cancer pain. *Adv. Neurol.,* **4,** 707

49 Levin, A. B., Benson, R. C. and Katz, J. (1978). Treatment of diffuse metastatic cancer pain by stereotaxic chemical hypophysectomy. Long term results and observations on mechanism of action. In *Pain Abstracts.* Vol. 1. p. 293. (Seattle: Int. Assoc. Study Pain)

50 Lipton, S., Miles, J. B. and Williams, N. E. (1979). Pituitary injection of alcohol for inoperable or intractable cancer pain. In Bonica, J. J. *et al.* (eds.). *Advances in Pain Research and Therapy.* Vol. 3, pp. 905–909 (New York: Raven Press)

51 Martino, C. and Ventafridda, V. (1978). Pain modulation in advanced breast cancer. In *Pain Abstract.* Vol. 1. p. 294. Second World Congress on Pain. (Seattle: Int. Assoc. Study Pain)

52 Hitchcock, E. and Leece, D. (1967). Somatotopic representation of the respiratory pathways in the cervical cord of man. *J. Neurosurg.,* **27,** 320

53 Lin, P. M., Gildenberg, P. L. and Polakoff, P. P. (1966). An anterior approach to percutaneous lower cervical cordotomy. *J. Neurosurg.,* **25,** 553

54 Crue, B. L. and Todd, E. M. (1964). A simplified technique of sacral rhizotomy for pelvic pain. *J. Neurosurg.,* **21,** 835

55 Sourek. K. (1977). Mediolongitudinal myelotomy. *Prog. Neurol. Surg.,* **8,** 15

56 Lambcke, R. (1964). Uber die mediolongitudinale chordotomie in Halsmakbereich. *Zentbl. Chir.,* **89,** 439

57 Hitchcock, E. (1970). Stereotactic myelotomy. *J. Neurol. Neurosurg. Psychiatr.,* **33,**

58 Hitchcock, E. (1977). Stereotactic spinal surgery. International Congress series 433. pp. 271–280. (Amsterdam: Exerpta Medica)

59 Schvarez, J. R. (1976). Stereotactic extralemniscal myelotomy. *J. Neurol. Neurosurg. Psychiatr.*, **39**, 53

60 King, P. B. (1977). Anterior commissurotomy for intractable pain. *J. Neurosurg.*, **47**, 7

61 Cook, A. W. and Kawakami, K. (1977). Commissural myelotomy. *J. Neurosurg.*, **47**, 1

62 Eiras, J., Garcia, J., Gornaz, J,. Carcavilla, L. and Ucar, S. (1981). First results with extra lemniscal myelotomy (E.M.) In Proceedings of the 4th meeting of the European Society for Stereotactic and Functional Neurosurgery. *Acta Neurochir.* (In press)

63 Zorub, D. S., Nashold. B. S. and Cook. W. A. (1974). Avulsion of the brachial plexus. 1. A review with implications of the therapy of intractable pain. *Surg. Neurol.*, **2**, 347

64 Nashold, B. S. and Ostdahl, R. H. (1981). Dorsal root entry zones lesions for pain relief. In Proceedings of Fourth meeting of the European Society for Stereotactic and Functional Neurosurgery. *Acta Neurol.* (In press)

65 White, J. C. and Sweet, W. H. (1979). Antero-lateral cordotomy. Open vs closed. Comparison and end results. In Bonica, J. J. *et al.*, (eds.). *Advances in Pain Research and Therapy.* Vol. 3, pp. 911–919. (New York: Raven Press)

66 Tasker, R. R. (1976). The merits of percutaneous cordotomy over the open operation. In Morley, T. P. (ed.) *Current Controversies in Neurosurgery.* p. 496–501. (New York: W. B. Saunders Company)

67 Hitchcock, E. (1973). Stereotaxic pontine spinothalamic tractotomy. *J. Neurosurg.*, **39**, 746

68 White, J. C. (1976). Role of sympathectomy in relief of pain. *Prog. Neurol. Surg.*, **7**, 131

69 White, J. C. and Sweet, W. H. (1969). *Pain and the Neurosurgeon. A Forty Year Experience.* (Springfield: C. C. Thomas)

70 Hupert, C. (1968). Recognition and treatment of causalgic pain occurring in cancer patients. *Pain Abstracts.* Vol. 1, p. 47. Second World Congress on Pain. (Seattle: Int. Assoc. Study of Pain)

71 Campbell, J. A. and Long, D. (1976). Peripheral nerve stimulation in the treatment of intractable pain. *J. Neurosurg.*, **45**, 692

72 Nashold, B. S. (1976). Electrical stimulation for pain relief. In *Current Controversies in Neurosurgery.* pp. 502–509. (New York: W. B. Saunders)

73 Long, D. M. (1978). Stimulation of peripheral nerves, spinal cord and brain for pain relief. In Swerdlow, M. (ed.). *Relief of Intractable Pain.* 2nd edn. (Amsterdam: Elsevier/North-Holland Biomedical Press)

74 Urban, B. J. and Nashold, B. S. (1978a). Percutaneous epidural stimulation of the spinal cord for relief of pain. *J. Neurosurg.*, **48**, 323

75 Urban, B. J. and Nashold, B. S. (1978b). Percutaneous epidural stimulation of the spinal cord. Technique and complications. In *Pain Abstracts.* Vol. 1, p. 297. Second World Congress on Pain. (Seattle: Int. Assoc. Study Pain)

76 Black, P. and North, R. (1978). Experience with spinal epidural electrical stimulation for intractable pain. In *Pain Abstracts.* Vol. 1, p. 296. 2nd World Congress on Pain. (Seattle: Int. Assoc. Study of Pain)

77 North, R. B. and Long, D. M. (1978). Epidural dorsal column stimulation for chronic intractable pain. 21 month follow up. In *Pain Abstracts.* Vol. 1, p. 296. Second World Congress on Pain. (Seattle: Int. Assoc. Study of Pain)

78 Adams, J. E., Hosobuchi, Y. and Fields, H. L. (1974). Stimulation of internal capsule for relief of chronic pain. *J. Neurosurg.*, **41**, 740

79 Mazars, G., Merienne, L. and Cioloca, C. (1979). Effets des soi-disant stimulations de la substance grise peri-acqueductale. *Neurochirurgie,* **25,** 96

80 Cosyns, P. (1978). Management of severe chronic pain in human by electrical central stimulation. *Pain Abstracts.* Vol. 1, p. 76. Second World Congress on Pain. (Seattle: Int. Assoc. Study of Pain)

81 Gybels, J., Dom, R. and Cosyns, P. (1979). Electrical stimulation of the central gray for pain relief in human: autopsy data. Proceedings of the 4th Meeting of the European Society for Stereotactic and Functional Neurosurgery. *Acta Neurochir.,* (In press)

82 Meyerson, B. A., Boethius, J. and Carlsson, A. M. (1979). Alleviation of malignant pain by electrical stimulation in the periventricular periaqueductal region. Pain relief as related to stimulation. In Bonica, J. J. *et al.* (eds.). *Advances in Pain Research and Therapy.* Vol. 3, pp. 525–533 (New York: Raven Press)

83 Ray, C. D. and Burton, C. V. (1979). Deep brain stimulation for severe chronic pain. Proceedings of 4th Meeting of European Soc. for Stereotactic and Functional Neurosurgery. *Acta Neurochir.* (In press)

84 Hosobuchi, Y. (1979). The current status of brain stimulation. In Proceedings of the 4th Meeting of European Society for Stereotactic and Functional Neurosurgery. *Acta Neurochir.,* (In press)

85 Richardson, D. E. and Akil, H. (1977). Pain reduction by electrical stimulation in man. Part 2: Chronic self administration in the periventricular gray matter. *J. Neurosurg.,* **47,** 184

86 Meyerson, B. (1979). European co-operative study on deep brain stimulation for pain. Resumé of the 3rd European Workshop on Electrical Neurostimulation.

87 Nashold, B., Slaughter, D. G., Wilson, W. P. and Zorub, D. (1977). Stereotactic mesencephalotomy. *Prog. Neurosurg.,* **8,** 35

88 Richardson, D. E. and Akil, H. (1975). A possible explanation for the effect of acupuncture on pain. *Confin. Neurol.,* **37,** 119

89 Watkins, E. S. (1978). The place of neurosurgery in the relief of intractable pain. In Swerdlow, M. (ed.) *Relief of Intractable Pain.* 2nd edn. (Amsterdam: Elsevier/North-Holland Biomedical Press)

90 Rodriguez-Burgos, F., Ajona, V. and Rubio, E. (1975). Stereotactic cryo-thalamotomy for pain. In Sweet, W. H., Obravor, S. and Martin Rodriguez, J. G. (eds.). *Neurosurgical Treatment in Psychiatry, Pain and Epilepsy.* pp. 679–683. (Baltimore: University Park Press)

91 Laitinen, L. V. (1975). Pulvinotomy for chronic pain. In Sweet, W. H., Obrador, S. and Martin Rodriguez. J. G. (eds.). *Neurosurgical Treatment in Psychiatry, Pain and Epilepsy.* pp. 669–672. (Baltimore: University Park Press)

92 Richardson, D. E. (1967). Thalamotomy for intractable pain. *Confin. Neurol.,* **29,** 139

93 Richardson, D. E. (1974). Thalamotomy for control of chronic pain. *Acta Neurochir.,* **21,** 77

94 Yoshi, N., Kudo. T. and Shimizu, S. (1973). Clinical and experimental studies of thalamic pulvinotomy. In *Abstracts of the Sixth Symposium of the International Society for Research in stero-encephalotomy.* Oct. 12–13. Tokyo.

95 Bouchard, G., Mayangi, G. and Martins, C. F. (1975). Advantages and limits of intracerebral stereotactic operations for pain. In Sweet, W. H., Obrador, S. and Martin-Rodriguez, J. G. (eds.). *Neurosurgery and Treatment in Psychiatry, Pain and Spasticity.* pp. 693–697. (Baltimore: University Park Press)

96 Hitchcock, E. (1973). Small frontal lesions for intractable pain. *Prog. Neurol. Surg.,* **8,** 114

97 Kuroda, R., Koshino, K., Kanai, K., Hayakawa, T., Kamikawa, K. and Mogamitt, . (1978). Anterior cingulamotomy for intractable pain relief. In *Pain Abstract.* Vol. 1. Second World Congress on Pain. (Seattle: Int. Assoc. Study Pain)

7

Current views on non-invasive methods in pain relief

M. Mehta

The management of a patient with chronic pain may present difficulties either because the pathogenesis of the underlying disease is uncertain and corrective measures directed at the source cannot be applied, or because there is inadequate response to available treatment. Ablative procedures, whether by surgery or neurolytic injection, do not necessarily relieve pain and may be followed by unacceptable neurological complications. The physician is therefore forced to rely on analgesic and allied drugs, but there are recognized limitations to their long-term use particularly when the patient has a normal life expectancy. Consequently the concept of stimulation or recruitment of inhibitory systems, proposed in the gate theory of Melzack and Wall[1] has attracted a great deal of interest even if significant improvement is obtained in less than 50% of cases. Fortunately most of the techniques applied at the *periphery* are relatively simple and trouble-free and even a modest improvement means less reliance on potent analgesic drugs. A *central* approach is necessary when dealing with an essentially subjective experience which does not rely entirely on peripheral sensory input[2]. The dominance of mind over matter has been recognized for many years and is reinforced by recent discovery of the internal opiates, encephalins and endorphins, released by the brain in the control of pain behaviour. Table 1 lists some of these central methods which have been underestimated in the past[3].

Table 2 lists some of the complex problems for which non-invasive methods of pain treatment may be indicated. It is based on the work of Merskey and his colleagues[4].

The Therapy of Pain

Table 1 Non-invasive methods of pain relief

I.   PERIPHERAL
      Stroking, rubbing, massage
      Counter-irritation and pain relieving sprays
      Vibration and percussion
      Trigger points + referred pain
      Physical methods (manipulation – traction – SW diathermy – ultrasonics)
      Neuromodulation by electric stimulation
      Acupuncture

II.   CENTRAL
      Cultural – religious – environmental
      Mental training and biofeedback
      Psychotherapy and hypnosis

IV.   NEOPLASTIC (adjunct to drugs, nerve blocks or cordotomy)
V.   CHRONIC INFLAMMATORY (e.g. chronic pancreatitis: post-encephalitis)
VI.   PSYCHIATRIC DISORDERS (anxiety, depression, neurosis, hysteria)
VII. PAIN OF UNKNOWN ORIGIN (e.g. restless leg syndrome; carotidynia)

Reprinted by permission. Copyright Spectrum Publication Inc. New York.

Table 2 Complex pain problems (for which non-invasive methods of pain treatment may be needed).

I.   MUSCULOSKELETAL
      1. Low back pain (e.g. spondylitis, arthritis, failed surgery)
      2. Chronic neck pain (cervical spondylosis, arthritis)
      3. Myofascial problems (e.g. frozen shoulder)
      4. Paget's disease or ankylosing spondylitis (with bony encroachment on nerves)
      5. Arthritis (rheumatoid, osteoarthritis, temperomandibular)

II.   NEUROLOGICAL
      1. Persistent headache
      2. Complex orofacial pains
      3. Central pain syndromes (e.g. thalamic or following a CVA)
      4. Neuralgias (e.g. trigeminal or postherpetic)
      5. Neuritis (e.g. diabetic, alcoholic or following trauma and neurolytic injections)
      6. Nerve lesions – (e.g. neuroma or nerve entrapment coccydynia and amputation stump pain)
      7. Causalgia and phantom limb pain
      8. Spasticity
      9. Neurological diseases (e.g. multiple sclerosis – tabes dorsalis)

III. AUTONOMIC
      1. Peripheral vascular disease
      2. Ischaemic cardiac pain
      3. Reflex sympathetic dystrophies (algodystrophies)

The table is based on the work of Merskey, from Smith, Merskey and Gross: *Pain Meaning and Management* (1979). Chapter 11.

172

I – PERIPHERAL NON-INVASIVE METHODS

Stroking: rubbing: massage: counter-irritation

Melzack and Wall's gate theory shifted the emphasis in pain therapy from drugs and ablative procedures to stimulation of myelinated nerve fibres for inhibition of pain transmission. It is illustrated by the way an animal licks an injured part and a child gains comfort from rubbing a smacked hand. The principle is extended to stroking, rubbing, massage and counter-irritation with icebags and pain relieving sprays. Nathan and Wall in their study of patients with post-herpetic neuralgia[5], emphasize the value of these simple remedies and insist on their trial before resorting to more complicated methods. Improvement is seldom dramatic or complete, as it is for example after a nerve block, and it is usually necessary for the patient to persist for at least a week before improvement is noticeable. In elderly and anxious individuals reinforcement, with a tricyclic antidepressant like amitryptiline is also indicated. These methods are particularly applicable to neuromuscular and joint pains which have not settled with rest and simple analgesics.

Vibration and percussion

These are further examples of the same basic principle. Percussion with a rubber hammer directed at the precise area of discomfort is initially very painful but a well-tried and effective treatment in some cases of pain, notably that due to neuromas occurring in an amputation stump[6]. Swerdlow[7], in an extensive trial, prefers a simple hand held vibrator and believes it is important for treatment to be directed accurately over the neuroma. This may be excruciatingly painful especially during the preliminary sessions, but patients will tolerate vibration if a tourniquet is first inflated over the upper part of the arm or thigh above the affected area. After a few minutes sufficient numbness is experienced for treatment to be tolerated. Vibration is recommended for 15–20 minutes, three or four times a day. Vibration therapy may also be helpful in localized muscle spasm causing persistent low back pain when a pad vibrator can be used, and in difficult cases of post-herpetic neuralgia.

Trigger points and referred pain

Brief, intense stimulation at accurately localized trigger points[8,9] can evoke disagreeable sensations both locally and at sites far removed from the source (see Figure 1). After transient discomfort long lasting pain relief may be achieved in this way. Impulses are generated by sharp

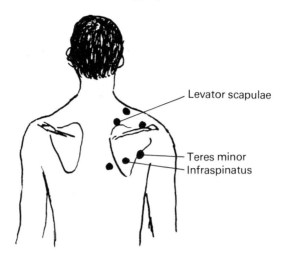

Figure 1 Common trigger points

digital pressure, repeated dry needling[10] injections of hypertonic saline or the application of cold sprays and counter-irritants. Acupuncture and transcutaneous electric stimulation, which will be described later, also seem to be effective in this way. Melzack *et al.*[11a] have shown that there is a marked correlation between acupuncture points and trigger points for pain. The stimulation caused by needling an acupuncture or trigger point may activate the descending inhibitory system. The same mechanism underlies many commonly unrecognized pain syndromes which can be treated effectively without resorting to unnecessary investigation or complicated therapy[11b]. These trigger areas appear to be zones of focal irritability, which are often myofascial in origin but exist in all tissues[12]. They are sometimes associated with definite nodules of fibrous tissue and may be sites of previous injury or disease. At these sites, just below the skin surface, there are small localized aggregations of nerve fibres and when these are stimulated they produce a low level of continuous afferent input into the central nervous system, inhibiting pain at the level of the 'gate' in the substantia gelatinosa. Detailed examination sometimes reveals patchy oedema and platelet aggregation associated with a surrounding area of intensive muscle spasm.

Trigger sites are detected by rucking up the skin, light touch, digital pressure or injections of 0.1–0.3 ml of hypertonic saline. Often a long and painstaking search is required to find these critical focal points. Pain relief is obtained by firm, rhythmic massage, injection of local anaesthetic, normal saline or topical application of cocaine. Ethyl chloride spray needs to be applied gently to produce an abrupt sensory stimulus but the treatment is ineffective if it is applied too vigorously and results in surface anaesthesia. A full range of passive, followed by active movements should be undertaken immediately afterwards.

Pain in the back of the head or neck, variously attributed to tension headache, whiplash injury or anxiety – hyperventilation, occurs in this way[13]. The symptoms are reproduced by localized pressure over the levator scapulae at the upper end of the scapula. Similarly a trigger point in the infraspinatus muscle accounts for pain in the shoulder extending down the arm. The pyriformis syndrome is interesting in that it frequently simulates how back pain with sciatica due to protrusion of an intervertebral disc. However there is no clinical evidence of nerve root tension or abnormal neurological signs and the critical point in diagnosis is pain reproduced by abduction and external rotation of the thigh against the pressure of the examiner's hand[9]. Further investigation and operative interference is clearly unnecessary in this case, because complete relief can be achieved by precise injection of the trigger zone in the pyriformis muscle with 2 ml of 1.5% lignocaine 20 mg of triamcinalone acetonide or 40 mg of methylprednisolone acetate (Depo-Medrone). Trigger points and referred pain are almost entirely confined to myofascial syndromes but are occasionally responsible for certain unusual neuralgias[8]. For example unilateral facial pain may emanate from focal irritation of the sphenopalatine ganglion. It can be elicited by pressure of a small gauze pack immediately over the ganglion, posterior to the proximal end of the middle turbinate bone. Facial pain and lachrymation from this source is often misinterpreted as toothache, migraine or sinus headache. The symptoms respond to topical application of 4% lignocaine or cocaine. Another unusual syndrome is fibrositic myofascial pain in intermittent claudication. In a recent publication Dorigo and his colleagues[14] find that local anaesthetic infiltration of trigger zones in the calf increases the exercise capacity of some patients with intermittent claudication. There is no improvement in regional blood flow, which suggests that focal areas of muscle irritation rather than an abnormal circulation are responsible for the chronic pain.

Physical methods of pain relief
Any discussion on non-invasive pain therapy would be incomplete without brief mention of physical methods, such as traction, manipula-

tion, mobilization and the application of heat or cold. Dry heat is given in the form of infrared for superficial heating and short wave for deeper penetration, as, for example, in arthritic joints. Moist heat is provided by hot packs or wax baths and may be particularly helpful in the treatment of painful conditions affecting the hand and feet. Ice packs or pain relieving sprays can be used to relieve pain after soft tissue injuries or due to arthritis of superficial joints. These are traditional methods available in the physiotherapy department and, although there can be no doubt of their practical value, their efficacy has not yet been exposed to controlled trials against analgesic drugs and other simple methods of treatment. Short-wave diathermy, together with intermittent traction, is recommended for pain due to cervical spondylosis which will not settle with diazepam and a collar worn at night[15]. Ultrasound is beneficial in the treatment of pain due to soft tissue injuries and may also be helpful in facial neuritis[16]. Ultrasonic radiation has also been stated to produce satisfactory results occasionally in amputation stump pain[17].

Neuromodulation by electric stimulation

Electricity's pain relieving potential was recognized by the early Egyptians and Hippocrates but its first recorded use was by the Roman physician, Scribonius Largus, in A.D. 46 when he treated gout and headaches by applying a torpedo fish known as the electric ray. Recent interest has been engendered by the gate theory and improvements in solid state electronics[18,19]. Electric stimulation modifies pain response partly by release of endogenous opiates in the vicinity of the midbrain and partly by recruitment of the inhibitory pathway in the substantia gelatinosa[20]. Consequently electric implants are probably more suitable for severe diffuse pain whereas transcutaneous stimulation, which is the main topic in this chapter, is indicated for localized, segmental pain of mild or moderate severity[21].

Transcutaneous electric stimulation (TNS) was used originally as a screening test for suitability of implanting an electrode on to a peripheral nerve or the dorsal columns of the spinal cord but this function has been superseded by direct stimulation[22]. However TNS has proved to be a useful therapeutic modality in its own right and control studies have shown that analgesia is not due entirely to a placebo effect[23]. Pain relief provided in this way is not immediate or complete, as it is after a nerve block. Patients and their relatives, impressed by what they have learned from friends or from advertisements, need to be suitably instructed to avoid disappointment. Nevertheless the technique is a relatively simple, trouble-free means of alleviating chronic pain in over 50% of a difficult group of patients who have not benefited from other methods. Some expect too much from it or find the sensations induced by electric stimulation more distressing than the original complaint. In a few cases initial improvement is not maintained because the subject accepts what has been achieved but focuses entirely on what remains. Consequently some authorities recommend a psychiatric analysis in addition to the usual range of investigations undertaken to determine the cause of pain[24]. Careful patient selection and instruction is an integral part of the technique.

The power source is a high output impedance generator with a spiked or square wave form and repetitive firing rate. There seems to be little significant difference between the numerous models available, provided they supply the essential parameters of electrical function[25]. Constant current, although less comfortable than constant voltage, is more effective and produces tingling in the area of pain. It is essential to search diligently for the optimum site of electrode application which produces this paraesthesia. Malleable carbon electrodes, or sponges suitably dampened beforehand, are moved around initially in the area of maximum discomfort or segmental distribution of the peripheral nerve involved. They are held in position or attached by tape but paint-on electrodes may be an improvement in this respect. Another innovation is a belt, incorporating a series of piezoceramic units, worn under the clothes. The output dial is turned on first and slowly increased until a regular thumping is felt in the requisite area. At this level of differential sensory excitation the current is not strong enough to evoke distressing muscle spasm or persistent dysaesthesiae. Next the rate is adjusted until the thumping is reduced to a mild tingle and finally the pulse width is adjusted, while the decreasing output, until the maximum comfort is achieved. Stimulation may be continuous or intermittent for periods up to quarter of an hour, which surprisingly may produce analgesia of many hours duration[26]. Opinions vary on the frequency and duration of electric stimulation but most clinicians agree that precise location of the sites is important. In the author's practice stimulation is carried out at the highest level which the patient can tolerate for approximately half an hour. After six of these sessions progress is reviewed and continuation of the technique discussed. Many patients can be instructed to use the apparatus at home when longer periods of stimulation can be performed. Some can anticipate the onset of pain, commonly in phantom limb or amputation stump disorders, and use the machine to minimize subsequent disagreeable sensations. Because of the initial placebo response most clinicians prefer not to make any decision on the effectiveness of the technique without a preliminary assessment of at least a month.

Transcutaneous electric stimulation is indicated for localized pain of mild or moderate intensity which has not responded to other measures. It is particularly useful for peripheral nerve injuries, localized arthritis, amputation stump and phantom limb pain[27,28]. Trigeminal and post-herpetic neuralgia may be treated in the same way[5] but the results are better, in the author's experience, if combined with psychotropic drugs[29]. Sympathectomy is the treatment of choice for causalgia but TNS is also effective[30]. There are also encouraging reports of its use in the difficult field of chronic low back pain[31] and for myofascial injuries, especially muscle tears and chronic ligamentous strains. Electric stimulation has been recommended for cancer and post-radiation pain but the results, in the author's practice, have been most disappointing. Brief periods of intense stimulation have been advocated for migrainous headaches and atypical facial neuralgia but pain relief is extremely variable. Indeed TNS has been tried empirically for any form of chronic pain, because it is easy to administer and relatively trouble free, but this practice should be discouraged unless every effort has been made to determine the underlying cause.

Electric stimulation is contraindicated for the emotionally unstable, psychoneurotic and those who are dependent on narcotic analgesics. Paraplegics, those with injuries to the brain and spinal cord or central pain states like thalamic pain, and individuals with backache due to adhesive arachnoiditis are unlikely to derive any benefit. Relative contraindications exist for those with demand pacemakers, contact dermatitis and pregnant women in the first trimester. The effects on diabetic neuritis and peripheral neuropathies are unknown. Electrodes should not be placed over the carotid sinus, particularly in those with nervous disposition. Complications are rare, presumably because such small electric currents are being used. Allergic skin eruptions due to contact materials and superficial burns may occur after repeated administrations but are uncommon.

Summary

The present consensus of opinion is that transcutaneous electric stimulation is not a panacea for all forms of intractable pain but it is a useful ad-

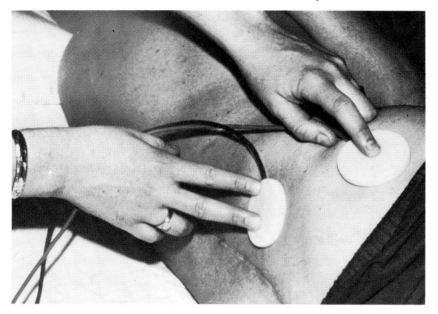

Figure 2 Transcutaneous electric stimulation (TNS) being used for the relief of intractable backache and sciatica

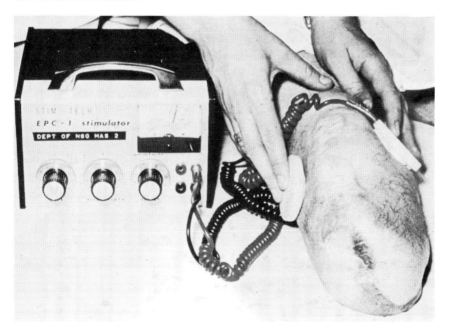

Figure 3 Transcutaneous electric stimulation (TNS) being used for relief of phantom limb pain

179

junct in many instances. It often enables symptoms to be better tolerated and reduces the need for strong analgesic drugs. Some older patients find it difficult to manage the apparatus or are fearful of its effects when they are alone. The cost of these machines is also a limiting factor but this can be overcome by loans from hospital departments or by charitable donations. Some firms will provide the equipment on renting or hire purchase terms and will usually repurchase it when the patient, after a genuine period of trial, finds it ineffective. The biggest disappointment, however, is the number of people who either expect too much or will not persevere with the treatment. Careful patient selection may well be the answer.

ACUPUNCTURE

Acupuncture has received a great deal of interest and publicity in recent years, following the visits of various medical delegations to China and other centres in the Far East, even though this traditional art has been practised for several centuries in the diagnosis and treatment of disease and suffering[32]. It has also been used as an alternative to conventional anaesthesia for surgery but the present account deals primarily with the role of acupuncture in the management of chronic pain. However the use and effectiveness of this technique has become a major controversy because of the wide variety of methods referred to as therapeutic acupuncture[33]. On the one hand there are a small number of highly trained traditional acupuncturists who use a complex Chinese system of diagnosis and treatment, while on the other, there are a much larger group who, with little or no previous knowledge, have adopted an entirely symptomatic approach to the subject. More recently electrical stimulation of the needles has been added to the empirical method and results in further divergent opinions regarding the best way to perform the technique. However there is no doubt acupuncture produces analgesia[34], even though it cannot be explained simply in terms of distraction, counter-irritation or even mass hypnosis[35, 36]. Presumably presynaptic inhibition is induced in the substantia gelatinosa and there may also be release of endorphins[37] or stimulation of the autonomic nervous system as contributory factors. It is also suggested that acupuncture is more effective in altering attitudes to pain than modifying the underlying disease[38]. Our present experience indicates that permanent analgesia is rarely achieved but it would be unwise to dismiss the technique because of this or because a complete scientific explanation is not readily available.

One definition of acupuncture is the application of certain stimuli on or through the surface of the skin in specific locations for the purpose of producing a local or systemic therapeutic response[33]. Thin, stainless steel needles (28 to 36 gauge) are commonly used. They vary considerably in length, shape and thickness but these are unimportant criteria. Many clinicians are happy to use ordinary 26 to 30 S.W.G. hypodermic needles, selecting short ones approximately one inch in length for surface areas on the head and face and longer three inch ones for more fleshy situations. There is minimal pain on initial impact but the exact site and depth to which the needles must be inserted are critical. It is a major assumption of acupuncture that certain areas of the skin are more sensitive to stimuli than other areas but the precise location of these acupuncture points or acupoints is based on a great deal of empiricism. Although there may be a correlation between these points, meridians and recognized dermatomes it is more likely that they indicate the position of localized subcutaneous nerve plexuses[39]. Brief, intense, stimulation gives rise to a characteristic feeling of dull ache, heaviness and paraesthesia ex-

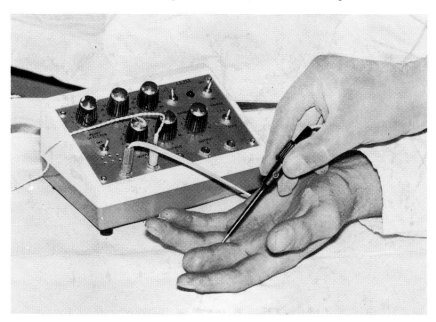

Figure 4 Electric acupuncture – detection of acupuncture points. The patient is holding the indifferent electrode in one hand (not seen in the picture), while the small exploring electrode is lightly pressed over the skin to detect a localized area of low electrical resistance. The acupuncture point is indicated by a sudden loud clicking sound.

tending some distance away from the point of needle insertion[40]. Pain relief is also obtained by dry needling[41], injection of hypertonic saline and application of cold sprays or transcutaneous electric stimulation at the same points. Nathan[34] notes that to be effective electric stimulation with an acupuncture needle needs to be strong enough to give repeated muscle contractions and believes that all motor points are acupoints but all acupoints are not necessarily motor points.

A standard acupuncture atlas[42,43] will show over 300 basic sites but there are other detailed methods of identification and acupuncture units of measurement[44]. In many instances the points coincide with areas of lowered electrical resistance compared with the rest of the skin surface. The subject holds the indifferent electrode while a small exploring electrode is lightly passed over the skin until a point of large electrical potential difference, indicating lowered skin resistance, is located by a sudden increased loud clicking sound. Insertion of the needle at the correct site is said to be critical to the success of the technique but most clinicians confine themselves to a number of simple tests. The author looks for tender spots or myofascial trigger points with deep finger pressure and confirms

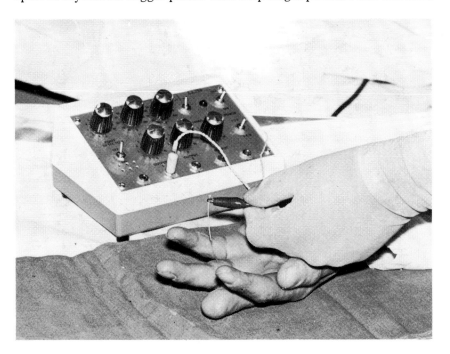

Figure 5 Electric acupuncture. Electric stimulation of the needle for the treatment of a patient with a painful neuroma in the finger

their location with an exploring electrode described already. Firm percussion or exploration with a needle point for points of hyperaesthesia in the periosteum is also recommended.

It is advisable to perform this technique under an aseptic regime and the author prefers to scrub his hands, clean the skin and use needles which have been stored in an appropriate antiseptic solution. The acupuncture point is determined by one of the methods described and confirmed by repeated up and down needle thrusts or 180° rotation in a clock-wise manner eliciting a 'gripping' sensation or the characteristic radiating paraesthesia. Further stimulation is conducted in a number of ways. Some twist the needles manually or move it vertically by means of an electrically operated holder. Others are content to have the needles in place without stimulation for 5–30 minutes. The author prefers electric stimulation for half an hour. Figures 3 and 4 show a suitable machine for this purpose, combining a sensitive galvanometer for detection of acupuncture points together with a series of electric circuits, employing varying parameters for subsequent intense stimulation. Slow waves of electric stimulation, up to 10 Hertz, seem to be less effective than faster ones at approximately 100 Hertz but a repeatedly changing rhythm may be the best of all[45]. The voltage is gradually increased in stepwise fashion to the limit of the individual's tolerance and maintained for about half an hour. At the conclusion of treatment the needles are slowly withdrawn, allowing time for associated muscle spasm to subside. Mann[42], in his extensive experience, emphasizes that not everybody responds to acupuncture. Ten per cent are positive reactors, recognized by their susceptibility to drugs and hypnotism and their low pain threshold. Probably a similar percentage do not react at all while the rest are variable in their response.

There are many other forms of stimulation. Some traditional acupuncturists use a lighted herb placed on the skin or on a thin strip of garlic or ginger root. The moxa herb is removed as soon as the patient experiences heat and thermal burns do not occur. Beneficial effects of moxibustion may be due to the herb as well as the intense stimulation. Transcutaneous electrodes, vibratory devices, ultrasonics, diathermy, infra-red or even laser beams are directed through small openings in heat-insulating covering materials such as asbestos. Infiltration or topical application of local anaesthesia nullifies the effect of acupuncture. A laser beam utilizes short focal length helium neon gas and exploits the ability of light at the red end of the spectrum to penetrate tissues[46]. It is used to detect acupuncture points and as a more convenient alternative to needling or electric stimulation in children, nervous adults and those in extreme pain. Early promising reports need to be confirmed by large scale controlled studies.

The exact position of acupuncture in pain relief is still under consideration. Many studies highlight the difficulties of unbiased assessment of an unconventional technique and measurement of a largely subjective experience like pain which has no reliable physiological index and is often embellished by emotional overtones[47]. Chapman with a psychophysical approach, believes the sensory aspects of pain are only slightly modified by acupuncture but, significantly the ultimate response of a patient is determined mainly by his attitude to the technique[48]. However most clinicians[49,50] believe it has more than a placebo effect and would recommend its use once the diagnosis is known and pain is unrelieved by more conventional methods. The empiric use of acupuncture cannot be condoned because temporary relief of pain and dysaesthesia may delay the recognition and treatment of a serious disease like chronic inflammation or cancer. Favourable responses have been noted particularly in the amelioration of musculoskeletal conditions, like long-standing muscle and ligamentous strains, intractable backache with sciatica, headache and various neuralgias. The author has used acupuncture to provide analgesia of more than six months duration in a few patients with trigeminal neuralgia, unrelieved by carbamazepine (Tegretol) and with neuromas following accidental injury which could not be treated in any other way. Pain relief is seldom complete and it seems that acupuncture often serves mainly as well as a useful adjunct to other methods.

There are isolated reports of sudden relief in pain of central origin, such as hemiplegia and thalamic pain of visceral origin due for example to peptic ulceration but a placebo effect cannot be discounted. A trial of acupuncture as a relatively uncomplicated method of pain relief in cancer pain may also be worthwhile particularly if repeated needling stimulates autoimmune mechanisms of the body. Provided it is carefully performed there are few complications from acupuncture. Broken needles due to abrupt withdrawal before associated muscle spasm has worn off, perforation of a viscus or pneumothorax and jaundice may occur, but these isolated reports do not indicate the status or training of the practitioner or the circumstances in which treatment was performed. Indeed the future of acupuncture is undecided because there are too few hard data to justify unequivocal judgement. In the author's view its main role appears to be as an adjunct to other methods in chronic pain states when conventional treatment has been unsuccessful.

II CENTRAL METHODS

Cultural: religious: environmental

Pain is unique amongst all sensory phenomena in that it is controlled primarily by the brain. Consequently the importance of mental training to subjugate the effects of physical and emotional trauma has been recognized for a long time. It is the basis of oriental cultures, such as Yoga and Transcendental Meditation, and explains the ability of the Indian fakir to lie on his bed of nails. This approach is more widely developed in underdeveloped countries where medical resources are limited, and mass indoctrination, as in China, is a relatively inexpensive way of enabling a large number of poor people to endure a variety of painful disabilities. The Chinese introduce this concept to children at school age and there may be a case, even in more affluent societies, for teaching the same principles to selected groups who are liable to be injured or in pain in an isolated or hostile environment. Any means of controlling severe pain, even temporarily, may be extremely useful when conventional medical aid is not immediately forthcoming[3]. In this context one thinks of the armed forces, policemen, explorers and missionaries who are extremely vulnerable in this way. Central pain control is more easily learned when the subject is provided with sufficient detailed information to recognize the intensity of peripheral stimulation and its modification by his own efforts[51]. This is the principle underlying autogenous *biofeedback*[52]. Recording systems are available for pulse rate, blood pressure, temperature, muscle activity and other parameters which influence the intensity of pain. It may take several sessions to learn the technique and eventually master the symptoms without relying on a monitor but biofeedback may have an important part to play in the management of migraine, tension headache, and pain associated with muscle spasm. Zitman[53] in a review of biofeedback training in patients with chronic pain, believes it is not superior to simple relaxation procedures, which are equally effective but less complicated and expensive to institute.

Pain is often, but not exclusively, due to an organic disturbance but there is a danger of the clinician becoming too preoccupied with this aspect and overlooking or delaying recognition of concomittant underlying psychosomatic factors[54]. Emotional and physical components of the pain experience are often inextricably interwoven into the fabric of the symptom complex with the result that an entirely physical approach is bound to result in incomplete relief. Psychotherapy is discussed in greater detail in chapter 2 but the general physician, surgeon or anaesthetist treating a pain patient often has to avail himself of many of these techniques apart from insight psychotherapy, which requires a considerable experience and some additional training[55].

Hypnosis

Hypnosis is another technique which is often of considerable help to pain workers who are not trained psychiatrists. This is an induced trance-like state in which suggestions are more readily accepted and acted on than is normally the case. The subject is not asleep and does not lose consciousness, even if he is less critical of his environment and unable to reject ideas or proposals put before him[56]. By fully engaging the conscious mind, less dominant areas of the brain are uncovered and memories of events long since forgotten, are brought into focus. This may enable him to put into perspective important activating factors which are causing or accentuating the pain. In addition it teaches a patient to relax, increase his pain tolerance and diminish his dependence on patent analgesic drugs. On one occasion it significantly helped a patient with multiple sclerosis to accept his pain and disabilities without continued prescription of narcotic analgesics[57].

Yoga and transcendental meditation

There is undoubtedly a significant psychosomatic basis to chronic pain, accentuated by the emotional strains and anxieties of modern living. Yoga and Transcendental Meditation teach an individual to relax, physically and mentally, and concentrate on matters other than physical illness. In Yoga the subject is taken through stages of abstention, observance, posture, breath control, sense withdrawal, concentration, meditation and contemplation. When fully trained the patient can withstand considerable sensory disturbance and this may be of considerable help in conditions like amputation stump and phantom limb pain.

Autosuggestion: Christian Science and Spiritual Healing

Autosuggestion is a form of self-hypnosis, potentially dangerous in those with an intense, vivid and uncontrolled imagination. Christian Scientists believe all pain and suffering can be alleviated by a positive attitude of self-confidence and deliberate exclusion of morbid preoccupation with disease. By refusing to accept medical advice, they may unnecessarily delay the early recognition and treatment of pain. The General Medical Council has recently officially recognized Spiritual Healing but the laying on of hands, often without the individual concerned being present, relies a great deal on mass hysteria and possibly autosuggestion or even spontaneous remission of the symptoms.

References

 1 Melzack, R. and Wall, P. D. (1965). Pain mechanisms: a new theory. *Science N.Y.*, **150,** 971
 2 Hannington-Kiff, J. (1974). *Pain Relief.* (London: William Heinemann)
 3 Mehta, M. (1978). Alternative methods of treating pain. *Anaesthesia*, **33,** 258
 4 Merskey, H. (1978). Diagnosis of the patient with chronic pain. *J. Human Stress*, **4,** 2
 5 Nathan, P. W. and Wall, P. D. (1974). Treatment of post-herpetic neuralgia by prolonged electric stimulation. *Br. Med. J.*, **3,** 645
 6 Russell, W. R. and Spalding, I. M. K. (1950). Treatment of a painful amputation stump. *Br. Med. J.*, **2,** 68
 7 Swerdlow, M. (1979). Personal communication.
 8 Travell, J. (1976). Myofascial trigger points: clinical view. In Bonica, J. J. and Albe-Fessard, D. (eds.). *Advances in Pain Research and Therapy*, Vol. 1, p. 919. (New York: Raven Press)
 9 Simons, D. G. (1976). Muscle pain syndromes. *Am. J. Phys. Med.*, Part I, **54,** 289–209. Part II, **55,** 15–43
10 Lewit, K. (1979). The needle effect in relief of myofascial pain. *Pain*, **6,** 1, 83
11a Melzack, R., Stilwell, D. M. and Fox, E. T. (1977). Trigger points and acupuncture points for pain; correlations and implications. *Pain*, **3,** 3
11b Pace, J. B. (1975). Commonly overlooked pain syndromes responsive to simple therapy. *Postgrad. Med.*, **58,** 107
12 Wyant, G. M. (1979). Chronic pain syndromes and their treatment. II Trigger points. *Canad. Anesth. Soc. J.*, **26** 3, 216
13 Sola, A. E. and Kuitert, J. H. (1955). Myofascial trigger point pain in neck and shoulder. *Northwest. Med.* (Sept.) 980
14 Dorigo, B., Bartolt, V., Grisillo, D. and Beconi, D. (1979). Fibrositic myofascial pain in intermittent claudication. Effect of anaesthetic block of trigger points on exercise tolerance. *Pain*, **6,** 180
15 Kay, N. R. M. (1977). Pain in the neck and arms. *Hosp. Update*, (March), 121
16 Antropa, M. (1974). Use of ultrasonics in facial nerve neuritis. *Zh. Nevropatol Psikhiatr.*, **74,** 506
17 Sutherland, S. (1978). *Nerves and Nerve Injuries.* 2nd edn. p. 452. (London: Churchill Livingstone)

Electric stimulation

18 Long, D. M. (1974). Cutaneous afferent stimulation for relief of chronic pain. *Clin. Neurosurg.*, **21,** 257
19 Shealey, C. N. (1974). Transcutaneous electric stimulation for control of pain. *Clin. Neurosurg.*, **21,** 269
20 Liebeskind, J. C., Mayer, J. C. and Akil, H. (1974). Central mechanisms of pain inhibition studies of analgesia from focal brain stimulation. In Bonica, J. (ed.). *Advances in Neurology*, Vol. 4, pp. 261–268. (New York: Raven Press)
21 Long. D. and Hagfors, N. (1975). Electric stimulation in the nervous system: The current status of electric stimulation of the nervous system for relief of pain. *Pain*, **1,** 109
22 Long, D. M. (1977). Electric stimulation for the control of pain. *Arch. Surg.*, **112,** 884

23 Long, D. M. and Carolan, M. T. (1974). Cutaneous afferent stimulation in the treatment of chronic pain. In Bonica, J. (ed.). *Advances in Neurology*, Vol. 4, pp. 755–759. (New York: Raven Press)

24 Shealey, C. N. and Maurer, D. (1976). Transcutaneous nerve stimulation for control of pain. *Surg. Neurol.*, 2, **1,** 45

25 Glynn, C. J. (1977). Electric stimulation for pain relief. *Br. J. Clin. Equip.*, **2,** 184

26 Melzack, R. (1975). Prolonged relief of pain by brief, intense transcutaneous somatic stimulation. *Pain*, **4,** 357

27 Miles, J. and Lipton, S. (1978). Phantom limb pain treated by electric stimulation. *Pain.* **5,** 373

28 Sternbach, R. A., Ignelzi, R. J., Deems, L. M. and Timmerman, G. (1976). Transcutaneous electric analgesia: a follow-up analysis. *Pain*, **2,** 35

29 Taub, A. and Collins, W. F. (1974). Observations on the treatment of denervation dysaesthesias with psychotropic drugs. In Bonica, J. (ed.). *Advances in Neurology*, Vol. 4, pp. 309–315 (New York: Raven Press)

30 Meyer, G. A. and Fields, H. L. (1972). Causalgia treated by selective large fibre stimulation of peripheral nerves. *Brain*, **95,** 163

31 Rutkowski, B., Niedzialkowska, T. and Otto, J. (1977). Electric stimulation in chronic low-back pain. *Br. J. Anaesthesia.*, **49,** 629

Acupuncture

32 Mann, F. (1972). *Acupuncture, The Ancient Chinese Art of Healing.* 2nd Revised edn. (London: Heinemann Medical Books)

33 Rubin, P. (1977). Therapeutic acupuncture. A selective review. *Southern Med. J.*, **70,** 8, 974

34 Nathan, P. W. (1978). Acupuncture analgesia. *Trends in Neuro-Sciences* (T.I.N.S.), **2,** 21

35 Stewart, D., Thomson, J. and Oswald, I. (1977). Acupuncture analgesia; an experimental investigation. *Br. Med. J.*, **1,** 67

36 Murphy, T. M. and Bonica, J. J. (1977). Acupuncture analgesia and anaesthesia. *Arch. Surg.*, **112,** 896

37 Editorial (1978). Human beta-endorphin: The real opium of the people? *Br. Med. J.*, **2,** 155

38 Toomey, T. C., Ghia, J. N., Mao, W. and Gregg, J. M. (1977). Acupuncture and chronic pain mechanisms: the moderating effects of affect, personality and stress on response to treatment. *Pain*, **3,** 137

39 Khong, T. K. (1976). Acupuncture in the relief of pain. A review. *Pharmatherapeutica*, **1,** iii

40 Melzack, R., Stillwell, D. and Fox, E. (1977). Trigger points and acupuncture points for pain. Correlations and implications. *Pain*, **3,** 3

41 Lewit, K. (1979). The needle effect in relief of myofascial pain. *Pain*, **6,** 1, 83

42 Mann, F. (1977). Acupuncture. In Lipton, S. (ed.) *Persistent Pain – Modern Methods of Treatment*, Vol. I, pp. 101–112 (London: Academic Press)

43 Mann, F. (1966). *Atlas of Acupuncture – Points and Meridians in Relation to Surface Anatomy.* (London: William Heinemann)

44 Chaitow, L. (1976). *The Acupuncture Treatment of Pain.* (Wellingborough: Thorson Publishers)

45 Nathan, P. W. (1978). Personal Communication

46 Caspers, K. H. (1977). Laser stimulation in therapy. *Phys. Med. Rehabil.*, **18,** 9

47 Bonica, J. J. (1974). Therapeutic acupuncture in the People's Republic of China: implications for American medicine. *J. Am. Med. Assoc.*, **228,** 1554
48 Chapman, C. R. (1975). Psychophysical evaluation of acupuncture analgesia. *Anesthesiology,* **43,** 5, 501
49 Lee, P. K., Andersen, T. W. and Modell, J. H. (1975). Treatment of chronic pain with acupuncture. *J. Am. Med. Assoc.*, **232,** 1133
50 Yamauchi, N. (1976). The results of therapeutic acupuncture in a pain clinic. *Canad. Anesth. Soc. J.*, **23,** 196

Central

51 Finley, W. W., Niman, C., Standley, J. and Ender, P. (1976). Biofeedback and Self-Regulation, **1,** 169
52 Johnstone, D. (1978). Clinical applications of biofeedback. *Br. J. Hosp. Med.,* November, p. 561
53 Zitman, F. G. (1979). Review biofeedback training in patients with chronic pain. Communication to the Intractable Pain Society of Great Britain, Dublin.
54 Sternbach, R. (1974). *Pain Patients: Traits and Treatment.* (London: Academic Press)
55 Merskey, H. (1978). Psychological aspects of pain relief. In Swerdlow, M. (ed.) *Relief of Intractable Pain*, 2nd edn. pp. 21–48 (Amsterdam, New York, London: Excerpta Medica.)
56 Hilgarde, E. R. and Hilgard, J. R. (1975). *Hypnosis in Relief of Pain.* (Los Altos, California: Kaufmann)
57 Mehta, M. (1977). Different approaches to the management of pain. In *Pain – New Concepts in Measurement and Treatment.* p. 116. (Edinburgh: Churchill Livingstone)

8

Current views on the management of pain in the cancer patient

R. D. Hunter

INTRODUCTION

Clinical and experimental cancer research has enjoyed a tremendous increase in activity over the last decade. The main thrust has been towards an understanding of fundamental mechanisms of carcinogenesis, early detection and improved radical curative treatment. It remains a sad fact that the solid tumours that have long provided the bulk of the work load to specialists working within any clinical discipline have failed to respond to this increased effort and the real success stories of the last decade still belong with the rarer paediatric tumours, lymphomas and germ cell tumours.

The clinical problem of severe pain in patients with malignant disease represents only one facet of overall cancer management. The direct attention of clinical investigators is rarely addressed to this problem alone but inevitably many of the advances in diagnostic and therapeutic techniques developed for this field have implications for those managing the 'cancer' patient with pain. This chapter will consider how these improvements may be capable of aiding management and the hope they give of future benefits.

The cause of chronic pain in patients with malignant disease never changes. The growing cell population does not produce pain from within itself but from attack on normal tissues by the developing, invading tumour. From a practical point of view that means damage to bone, invasion of neurovascular bundles and pressure on peripheral nerves or their roots of origin. The non-specific nature of the symptomatology produced often leads to problems of diagnosis and may call for considerable acumen in assessment. Three important facts must always be borne in mind by anyone involved in managing these patients.

First the premise that 'unremitting pain associated with cancer is a late manifestation'[1] must be avoided. Patients with peripheral bronchogenic carcinoma fixed to the chest wall or invading the brachial plexus (Pancoast syndrome) have chronic unremitting pain which may prove difficult to assess non-invasively. They remain potentially curable surgically[2] and radiotherapeutically[3]. As a group, patients with this disease have a prognosis as poor as the whole group of patients with bronchogenic carcinoma[4] but they are not inevitably incurable even with existing techniques of assessment and management.

Secondly, the occurrence of chronic pain in a patient who has previously had treatment for malignant disease does not mean that it must be due to recurrent disease. Careful assessment of a group of patients with back pain after treatment for primary malignant disease allowed Galasko and Sylvester[5] to ascribe the symptoms to benign intercurrent disease in one third of patients. Unfortunately, for the majority of patients, the situation is less happy and the pain represents one further incident in a progressive illness of finite length, an important factor that must strongly influence the diagnostic and therapeutic techniques used with these patients.

Finally, pain even in the presence of active malignant disease, can be present for a variety of reasons. Though most patients symptoms are due to the tumour itself, mechanical instability due to skeletal destruction, secondary infection of a cavity, e.g. sinus or uterus or inflammation around the periphery of the tumour, can and do cause chronic pain[6]. This chapter will be concerned with pain due to active tumour.

DIAGNOSTIC TECHNIQUES

All investigations remain a poor substitute for a good history and clinical examination. To these and the standard radiological and biochemical investigations the last few years have added four techniques that can aid the identification or mapping of recurrent and metastatic cancer.

(1) Isotope scintigraphy (or isotope scanning)
(2) Ultra sonography
(3) CAT scanning
(4) Biochemical tumour markers

Unfortunately, only the last type of investigation results from a positive function of the tumour. The others are concerned with the detection of an abnormality in normal structure or function. The problem with this negative type of investigation often lies in the technical limitations of the equipment being used and calls for some understanding of these limitations when assessing any result that is not unequivocally positive.

Isotope scintigraphy

This branch of diagnostic radiology has benefited very fully in the last decade from technical improvements in scanning equipment, the development of gamma cameras, the very wide range of artificial radionuclides available commercially and a better understanding of the advantages of nuclide coupling with physiologically handled substances. As a result of these developments, organ imaging has improved dramatically both in speed and quality. For many patients with cancer, brain, liver, pancreas and spleen scanning provide important evidence about primary or metastatic disease.

For the patient in pain, only bone scanning represents a consistently useful investigation. The less practical radionuclides ^{18}F and ^{87}Sr have given way to bone scanning with ^{99m}Tc technetium phosphate complexes[7]. The abnormal scans (Figure 1) indicate an osteoblastic response of normal bone to attack by malignant disease and can precede diagnostic radiological changes by two years[8]. With experience false positive investigations can be satisfactorily eliminated[9]. False negative results can arise if a bony osteoblastic response is not mounted consistently, as e.g. in myeloma or at well recognized bony sites like the sacrum or pubis[10].

The investigation has proved sufficiently successful to replace the skeletal survey as the first investigation for detection of bony metastatic disease in patients with breast cancer[11]. For those with widespread disease it is useful as a relatively simple, inexpensive, non-invasive technique for mapping the extent of gross bony metastases and the general response of this disease to treatment[12].

One disappointing aspect of isotope scintigraphy in malignant disease has resulted from a critical appraisal of ^{67}Ga investigations[13]. This radionuclide was noted to localize a number of soft tissue tumours[14] and hopes of the first tumour specific localizing agent were high. Unfortunately, inflammatory lesions and normal organs have also been found to produce positive results[15] and recent co-operative lymphoma studies[16,17]

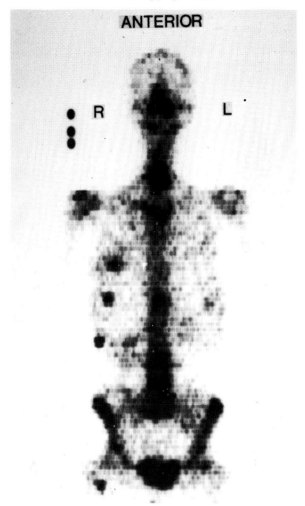

Figure 1 ^{99m}Tc polyphosphate whole body anterior bone scan in a patient presenting 2 years after mastectomy for carcinoma of the breast with diffuse bone pain and normal diagnostic X-ray films. The increased patchy uptake of isotope in the cervical and lumbar spine, right ribs and right humerus established the diagnosis of metastatic breast carcinoma. Reproduced by kind permission of Dr B. Eddleston, Christie Hospital

concluded that the technique is not sufficiently reliable for routine evaluation of extent of disease or response to treatment.

Ultrasonography
This relatively inexpensive technique, developed originally in obstetrics, has become much more widely available and found a useful role in many

clinical specialties. The development of modern ultrasound equipment with stored grey scale displays and 'real-time' scanners has contributed particularly to this advance.

In oncology the ability of the investigation to identify lymph node masses of 2–3 cm, particularly in the para-aortic region[18] and also to demonstrate pancreatic, retroperitoneal and pelvic masses[19.20] to monitor these quickly and non-invasively, and to study their response to treatment has commended further use and development. Much of the information obtained by this technique could otherwise only come easily from CAT scanning (see next section) but the relative cheapness and availability of ultrasound is an important factor influencing its use. The one real weakness of this approach is the importance of the skill of the operator and the quality of information obtained depends very much on this expertise. The technique is particularly useful in thin patients[21] and its place as an investigation of cancer patients suspected to have retroperitoneal or pelvic masses is evolving rapidly.

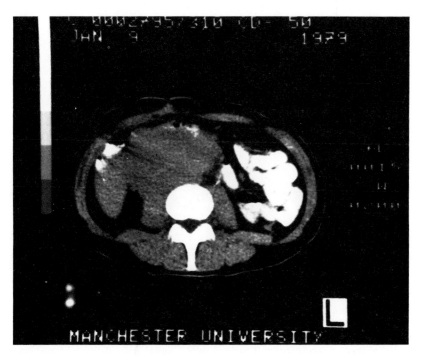

Figure 2 CAT scan of the para-aortic region in a patient with seminoma of the testes demonstrating a large soft tissue node mass anterior to the vertebral body on the right side and displacing the small bowel, displayed by contrast, to the left. Reproduced by kind permission of Professor I. Isherwood, Manchester University

CAT scanning

This highly sophisticated development of diagnostic radiology is already making an important impact on the management of patients with malignant disease[22]. The equipment, particularly the body scanner, is extremely expensive to buy and operate, is not widely available and, therefore, must only be used to obtain information that is not freely available from conventional, non-invasive diagnostic techniques.

To a patient in pain this technique can offer the accurate delineation of soft tissue masses at any site in the body and identify clearly the relationship between these and normal organs. This may be particularly useful when pain is arising from retroperitoneal tissues or the pelvis. Para-aortic (Figure 2) and internal iliac lymph node masses (greater than 2 cm) can

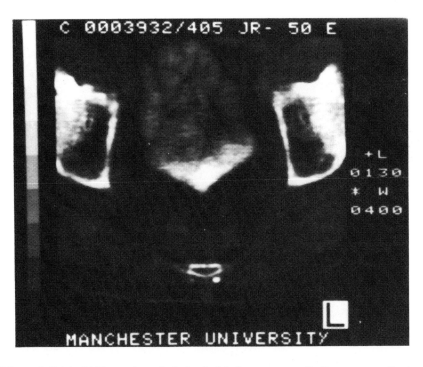

Figure 3 Pelvic CAT scan through the level of the lower sacrum. Radio-opaque media visible in small bowel in the midline. A soft tissue mass is present between the small bowel and the sacrum. The patient had had an AP resection for a rectal carcinoma 1 year previously. He complained of poorly localized perineal pain. Clinical and radiological investigations failed to achieve a satisfactory diagnosis but CAT investigation allowed local recurrence to be implicated and a successful course of X-ray therapy was given using this information about extent of disease. Reproduced by kind permission of Professor I. Isherwood, Manchester University

be identified[23], even in the presence of apparently normal lymphography, and their response to treatment assessed. The equally difficult problems of small retroperitoneal tumours[24] and recurrent adenocarcinoma of the kidney[22] can also be delineated. A final important development area has been the identification of bladder tumours and their metastases[25], recurrent rectal carcinoma (Figure 3) and the examination of the abdomen and pelvis in ovarian carcinoma[22].

The problem of identifying small or difficult bony metastatic disease has also been improved by this technique. Metastases in areas like the sacrum and pubis, which are poorly identified on conventional radiography and scintigraphy, can be identified when they are as small as 0.5 cm and osteoblastic. Equally important (cf. scintigraphy) pure osteolytic metastases 1–2 cm in size can also be visualized[22].

The technique again incorporates this important facility of monitoring the response of soft tissue disease (Figure 4) and bone metastases to

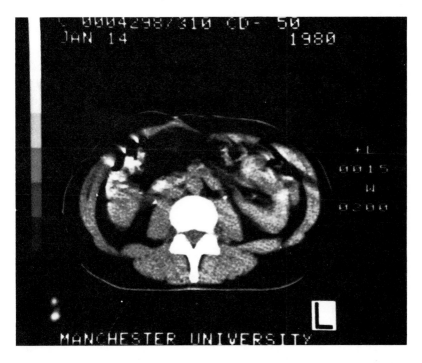

Figure 4 CAT scan at the same level on the patient shown in Figure 8.2 one year after X-ray therapy to the abdomen. The abnormal soft tissue mass has disappeared and the para-aortic region looks normal. Reproduced by kind permission of Professor I. Isherwood, Manchester University

197

treatment. For the radiotherapist the improved information from CAT scanning also offers the possibility of better treatment planning and, therefore, patient management.

For carefully selected patients this is probably the most important diagnostic development of the last few years.

Biochemical tumour markers

The identification of 'tumour marker' substances has been a useful aid to the assessment and management of some patients with malignant disease. A wide variety of substances are produced by human tumours and have been investigated using sensitive radioimmunoassay techniques. The aim of all these investigations has been to identify substances selectively produced by tumours. The best example is the rare choriocarcinoma in young women where assay of HCG in serum and urine allows an assessment of tumour burden, the response to treatment and the early identification of relapse[26]. The most widely used investigations are CEA (carcinoembryonic antigen) in large bowel[27] and breast cancer[28] and α-fetoprotein in germ cell tumours[29]. Dealing with a population of patients the techniques are not satisfactory as not all histologically similar tumours produce markers and the levels of marker substances produced do not invariably reflect the tumour burden.

The investigations can, however, have a useful place in the follow-up assessment of individual patients who have been shown, at the time of primary diagnosis, to have a marker-producing tumour. High or rising serum levels in such patients after primary radical treatment, particularly in those with vague or developing symptoms, can be shown to identify recurrent disease at an earlier stage[27,28] than by conventional techniques. For the patient with unidentified pain the demonstration of elevated or rising markers can, therefore, be a useful pointer to the diagnosis of tumour reactivity.

Conclusion

All of these investigations can only produce evidence to aid the assessment of the patient in pain. They are not all freely available and in view of this and the very different costs involved have to be used selectively and often sequentially. Bone scanning identifies only osteoblastic normal bone response to attack by malignant disease. Ultrasonography is useful in the identification of retroperitoneal and pelvic masses in thin patients. CAT scanning identifies the relationship of soft tissue masses to normal structures and can provide important information about the density of the mass under study. Between these three techniques the difficult clinical problems of pain arising from bone, the retroperitoneum and pelvis can be much more satisfactorily investigated. It is to be hoped that this improved diagnostic capability can aid patient management, as diagnosis in the absence of a therapeutic capability is of little value to the patient.

TREATMENT

Radiotherapy, surgery, hormone therapy and chemotherapy continue to play their individual parts in the management of malignant disease and the pain associated with it. All of these, along with the new technique of hyperthermia, will be discussed. These patients as a group have been a practical problem to radiotherapists for many decades and the clinical syndromes associated with pain in malignant disease and basic management techniques are well described[30].

Radiotherapy

No modality of treatment comes close to the speed and effectiveness of radiotherapy in the control of isolated deposits of malignant disease. In clinical practice palliative X-ray therapy continues to be used extensively and successfully in patients with pain from bony metastatic disease, lymph node masses and soft tissue disease infiltrating nerve plexuses and the chest wall. Chronic pain from attack on the axial skeleton by the common metastatic tumour represents the bulk of this workload.

Utilizing the best available diagnostic techniques for localization, some of which have been discussed above, megavoltage radiotherapy can be expected to relieve the pain of bony metastatic disease in 90% of patients treated[31]. This is seen even in patients with metastatic disease from so-called 'radio resistant tumours' and that concept should be ignored in this situation[32]. Successful palliation is maintained to death in the majority of patients achieving relief[33,34]. The mechanism by which only some bony metastases produce pain and the reason for the dramatic success of radiotherapy remain the subject of speculation[30,35].

Most radiotherapy centres employ a policy of giving tolerance doses of radiotherapy to localized pain producing deposits often over a number of days. Recent clinical studies[32–34] have confirmed two observations of Boland *et al.*[31] that must challenge this approach which is expensive both in patient and departmental time. Firstly, there is no evidence of a dose–response relationship between the dose of radiation and the response of the pain to treatment. Secondly, successful and maintained palliation of pain due to metastatic disease can be achieved by single doses of radiation that are well below normal tissue tolerances. These two important observations have, therefore, a number of practical and theoretical consequences.

The observation of the lack of relationship between dose of radiation and symptomatic response to treatment means that techniques designed to improve results of radical radiotherapy, e.g. neutron therapy, hypoxic cell sensitizers and sequential chemotherapy and radiotherapy, which are presently under intensive clinical study for radical treatment, can be expected to have no useful part to play in improving the management of painful bony metastatic disease. Megavoltage photon facilities are all that is required radiotherapeutically to treat these patients.

High dose tolerance radiotherapy of spinal metastatic disease is often accompanied by systemic upset and a temporary aggravation of symptoms. A more widespread adoption of a policy of relatively low dose single exposure radiotherapy deserves consideration for ambulant patients with bony metastatic disease. Since radiotherapy facilities tend to be centralized, treatment involves moving patients in pain sometimes considerable distances. This would therefore allow a simplicity of approach and reduce morbidity and would contribute to the quality of the life of patients whose quantity of life is well recognized to be determined by their extra skeletal metastases[36]. There would also be a considerable financial saving possible by avoiding or reducing the volume of in-patient treatment and cutting down fractionated therapy.

With the improved diagnostic techniques scintigraphy and CAT scanning available to map early metastatic bone disease, prophylactic irradiation of these areas has also emerged as an interesting new concept in bone pain management[35]. The possibility of using lower doses of radiation, as discussed above, would also allow larger volumes of bone to be included in any treatment. Such a policy of early intervention might be expected to reduce the physical destruction caused by progressing but asymptomatic metastatic disease. The pain from progressive spinal collapse due to this type of disease is unpredictable in its severity but inevitably the destruction will lead to spinal instability if the patient lives long enough. Surgical procedures are available to stabilize such a spine but a preventative policy based on early scanning and large field low dose radiotherapy deserves consideration in the slower moving varieties of disease, especially breast cancer.

Unfortunately, a policy of irradiating large volumes of bone with relatively low doses of radiation has some limitations. The bones involved in this type of metastatic disease contain the majority of the red marrow in adult patients[37] and irradiation of this can be expected seriously to impair marrow reserve. In the absence of any other active form of treatment an aggressive radiotherapy policy can be pursued but if chemotherapy is expected to play any part in the further management of the patient that marrow reserve cannot be allowed to be depleted and radiotherapy must be confined to symptomatic foci of disease.

The logical extension of a low dose extended field radiotherapy policy in patients with widespread symptomatic metastatic disease and for whom no other active treatment therapy is available, is whole body irradiation. Rider et al.[38] have recently described a well tolerated technique in which this is achieved by treating the patient in two separate halves (hemicorporeal) at 6 week intervals. Symptomatic responses, particularly pain relief, are claimed to be good with radiation lung tolerance emerging as the dose limiting factor[39,40]. Good responses have been claimed from patients with a wide variety of malignant disease.

Although the cause of bone pain in metastatic disease is unknown, the mechanism of the bone destruction of metastatic disease is now better understood. Osteoclast congregation, local tumour pressure and prostaglandin secretion[41,42] have all been implicated. X-ray therapy is indiscriminate in its damage and inevitably normal tissues, including osteoblasts and fibroblasts, share in the damage from radiotherapy given for deposits of metastatic disease[43]. These are tissues that will be required to heal the damaged bone after successful therapy and killing most of these cells with high dose therapy will inevitably weaken the tissues. One final attraction in a relatively low dose single exposure treatment policy is that a reduced amount of damage will be done to the important normal bone repair mechanisms. This would appear to be particularly important if pathological fractures have taken place or appear likely.

In contrast to the axial skeleton, the place of radiotherapy in the management of long bone metastatic disease is more difficult. With small symptomatic deposits, not threatening the integrity of the bone, local single exposure X-ray therapy is a simple solution. If primary surgery has fixed a fracture or excised a deposit the clinical problem becomes more complicated. The previously discussed damage to normal cell repair populations by X-ray therapy and the success of surgical fixation (see p. 203) encourages a slightly more cautious policy. No control studies have been carried out but clinical impression suggests that radiotherapy alone is a relatively poor modality for relieving pain in pathological fractures but in association with internal fixation usually given after surgery is thought to be more effective than fixation alone[44]. Perhaps one other factor that should be taken into account in making a final decision about X-ray therapy in patients treated surgically is the availability of an alternative form of active treatment, for example hormone or chemotherapy. Successful hormone manipulation or systemic chemotherapy will control local disease without such an adverse effect on local bone healing mechanisms as that caused by the X-ray therapy. If no such option is available then postoperative radiotherapy should be given or surgical fixation will prove only temporary due to local tumour progression.

Repeating X-ray therapy

With slowly progressing metastatic disease the radiotherapist is sometimes presented with the problem of considering re-treatment of a previously irradiated tumour deposit. The medical problem is complicated by the loss of long term tolerance of previously irradiated tissues and the fact that recurrence has taken place after the earlier success. Clinical experience suggests that only in a very sensitive tumour in a patient with a reasonable life expectancy should this policy be embarked on. It should be remembered that late radiation damage can produce very difficult management problems with very intense pain from tissue necrosis of neurological injury[45].

Whole body irradiation

Hemi-corporeal beam irradiation is not the only means whereby widespread bony metastatic disease causing intractable pain can be treated by radiotherapy. ^{32}P had been noted during the 1930s to be incorporated into growing tissue but the lack of differentiation of normal and abnormal tissue uptake had prevented its successful clinical use for many years[46]. The technique of androgen priming prior to administration of the radionuclide was reported to be successful in increasingly effective radionuclide uptake in tumours and remains in clinical use in relieving chronic pain from widespread bony metastatic disease. Satisfactorily maintained responses have been recorded in breast[47], prostate[46,48], and thyroid[49] carcinoma. The technique is technically simple requiring only a series of i.v. injections of the radionuclide but the androgen timing often aggravates pain[44] and the isotope can be profoundly toxic to the bone marrow.

More recently the radionuclide ^{89}Sr has been demonstrated to produce remarkable lasting relief of pain in a high proportion of selected patients with carcinoma of the prostate whose symptoms had not been controlled by X-ray therapy or hormone therapy. All patients had osteoblastic metastatic disease with high radionuclide uptake on scintigraphy. The isotope was injected[50] intravenously and early and maintained pain relief was observed. Unfortunately, the isotope is not freely available for this type of use and is expensive, but the simplicity of the technique and the lack of systemic or marrow toxicity strongly commends its urgent further assessment in this particular type of metastatic disease.

Surgery

While the symptoms of spinal metastatic disease can usually be controlled by X-ray therapy the problem of long bone deposits, particularly those in the commonest site, the femur, remain more complicated. The situation normally arises with carcinoma of the breast or bronchus but the whole spectrum of metastatic disease is evident in any large surgical series[51]. The observation that pathological fractures of large bones in patients with metastatic disease, usually from breast cancer, can slowly heal by immobilization[52] has revealed the paradox that bone attacked and destroyed by metastatic disease is still capable of a prompt, often exuberant, repair process[53]. This recognition has encouraged interested orthopaedic surgeons to pursue a much more active approach towards patients with pathological fractures, who can present a difficult nursing problem due to immobility and chronic pain unrelieved by analgesics. Active surgical intervention with internal fixation in patients with a life expectancy of more than a few weeks has been convincingly demonstrated to be successful in relieving this pain in over 80% of patients[51,54]. It is now even possible to resect local tumour and damaged bone replacing them with a prosthesis or internally fixing them and using a special cement[51]. Pain relief is the most consistent finding in these surgical series and in itself justifies the procedures. Of no less importance is the increased ease of nursing. Unfortunately, ambulation is not achieved as consistently as the relief of pain, but this in no way detracts from the usefulness of the procedure.

Success with pathological fractures has also encouraged a policy of prophylactic internal fixation in some patients[51,52,55]. Metastatic disease within the medullary cavity is not thought to be painful but increasing cortical destruction brings on pain[53]. Spontaneous fractures appear to occur in patients with more than 75% cortical involvement while minor trauma may cause fracture in those with above 50%[55]. Prophylactic fixation of progressing painful deposits with early cortical destruction can avoid emergency surgery in a traumatized and devitalized field. This policy is established in patients who have previously had a pathological fracture and who are recognized to have a high risk of further problems in other long bones. It deserves more active consideration among the general population of patients, especially those with breast cancer, whose painful metastatic disease in long bone can now be mapped and monitored (see the section on scintigraphy).

Although conservative surgery and radiotherapy palliate the majority of these patients with intractable pain from bony metastatic disease, slow progression of disease after treatment, fungation, and the presence of a rare solitary bone metastasis should still encourage the clinician to consider radical ablative surgery even if amputation is required in patients[56].

Hormone therapy

Hormonal therapy has maintained its place over the last few decades as a useful palliative form of treatment in patients with slowly progressive metastatic carcinoma, usually from carcinoma of the breast or prostate. Pain from bony metastatic disease is often a major problem although the presence of soft tissue recurrence, pleural or parenchymal lung deposits may also influence a treatment decision. Empiric observations of the objective and subjective responses of groups of patients to different endocrine ablative procedures or to a variety of synthetic hormone and antihormone preparations have allowed patterns of response to be established. This has, however, only defined in very general terms the patients who are likely to respond to a particular treatment. It has always been unsatisfactory clinically to know that a response rate of 20–40% is possible particularly when the ablative procedures, often determined by local expertise or enthusiasm, have carried with them the risk of increased postoperative morbidity and a requirement to consider long term chronic hormone replacement therapy. The operations of oophorectomy and orchidectomy carry little morbidity but adrenalectomy is a major operation requiring convalescence and hypophysectomy, even by cryosurgery, ^{90}Y implantation or alcohol injection, carries a significant risk of a devastating complication. Undoubtedly, the excellence of the results in patients who do respond to treatment have encouraged clinicians to continue using these procedures but the relatively low overall response rates have defied the use of clinical parameters in achieving better patient selection.

A major advance promises to place this type of treatment on a less empiric basis. Hormone receptors have been isolated biochemically in the cytoplasm and nucleus of human tissues, including cancers[57]. Starting with the receptors binding oestrogens in the cytoplasm of human breast cancer, the techniques have been expanded to demonstrate progestogen, androgen and glucocorticoid receptors in different tissues. The standardization of the assay procedures and a general consensus about the implication of these tissue receptors awaits the results of the intensive investigations which are currently underway.

Breast cancer remains the most studied and best understood clinical problem. Receptors have been demonstrated both in the cytoplasm[57] and nucleus[58] of human cancer and there has emerged an understanding of the complicated relationship of the cytoplasmic oestrogen and progestogen receptors and their influence on the nuclear oestrogen receptor.

More importantly the measurement of these receptors in human breast cancer has now established the prognostic value of such assay procedures[59]. The absolute receptor content can vary between primary and secondary deposits and between different types of deposit[60] at varying stages of the disease but the consensus opinion of the British workers[61] is that oestrogen receptor negative patients have only a 15% chance of responding to any type of hormonal therapy while cancers carrying receptors for oestrogen and progestogen have a 75% chance. When the more recently recognized nuclear receptors are taken into account, tumours showing no evidence of cytoplasmic or nuclear receptors have failed to show any response to hormonal therapy[62]. Substantiation of these findings could well completely alter the selection policy for therapy of advanced breast cancer and spare patients unnecessary treatment by eliminating those who have little or no chance of responding.

Similar investigations in prostatic carcinoma are at an earlier stage. Androgen receptors can be demonstrated in the cytoplasm of some human prostatic cancers[63]. Reasonable volumes of tissue are more difficult to obtain and the high endogenous androgen binding complicates the assays. Interestingly prostatic carcinoma also appears to carry an oestrogen binding receptor[64]. The limited clinical studies available at present have produced conflicting opinions[65,66] on the prognostic value of the hormonal patterns in determining the response to endocrine manipulation but it is hard to believe that when the technical problems are overcome the situation will not be similar to that demonstrated in breast carcinoma.

With improved patient selection emerging as a possibility the enormous advances of endocrinology in the last decade will open up some hope of a better understanding of the mode of action of hormonal therapy in human cancer. The inter-relationships of the hypothalamus, pituitary and the different endocrine end organs are complex but simple serum assay procedures and dynamic function tests now allow careful monitoring of endocrine function to be carried out without patient inconvenience, an important consideration for patients in considerable pain.

The confusion surrounding the present understanding of the place of ablative procedures in the control of pain from metastatic disease is best exemplified by considering the place of hypophysectomy. Using a wide range of ablative techniques patients with carcinoma of the prostate[67-69] and breast[70-72] in chronic pain due to metastatic bone disease have been shown to achieve dramatic and lasting relief of pain. Unfortunately, anatomical[73] and simple endocrinological studies[72,74,75] have failed to show any relationship between the degree of pituitary destruction and the relief of pain. No relationship is evident either in the response of measurable tumour and pain relief. The problem is made increasingly complicated by the experience of workers producing pituitary destruction and achieving pain relief in patients with metastatic carcinomas which are not responsive to endocrine manipulation[76-78].

The enormous experience of Moricca[76] substantiated by Lipton and his colleagues[77] indicates that two separate clinical experiments are being explored when pituitary damage is inflicted on a patient with metastatic carcinoma. The first is an endocrinological procedure and can be expected to produce remission of pain by a mechanism of tumour arrest or regression. The second is a poorly understood neurological lesion delivered to the pituitary or even the hypothalamus[73]. There is an urgent need to separate these two mechanisms by careful clinical experiment with accurate endocrinological and neurological assessment. The complications of a poor hypophysectomy – diabetes insipidus, meningitis, occular motor palsies and CSF rhinorrhea, when allied to the misery of widespread bone pain from metastatic disease are unacceptable to the majority of clinicians. However, the enormous increase in the quality of the patient's life when relief of pain is achieved demands this further assessment of these procedures.

From an endocrinological point of view the situation is changing again as anti-hormones in the form of anti-oestrogens, anti-androgens and anti-glucocorticoids have become widely available for clinical use in human cancer. It seems inevitable that drugs will become available which act as inhibitors of individual pituitary hormones and these will then allow a 'medical' hypophysectomy, particularly a selective hypophysectomy, to be studied at a clinical level without the risks of an invasive procedure. Improved patient selection, more sophisticated endocrine manipulation and more accurate neurological lesions should, within a few years, banish the mystique of hormonal therapy and spare many patients in pain from unsuccessful, unpleasant procedures.

Chemotherapy

For the patient whose malignant disease is widely metastatic only chemotherapy continues to offer even a theoretical possibility of cure. The majority of drugs available to interested physicians have been in use for at least a decade. They depend for their effect on killing the malignant cells (cytotoxicity) but they, like radiation, indiscriminately damage normal tissues as well as the malignant cell population. The drugs are usually administered systemically and what little specificity of action is seen clinically is due to concentration of the drug in an organ for pharmacological reasons.

Enormous numbers of studies have demonstrated the limited effectiveness of single chemotherapeutic agents in curative cancer therapy. This is thought to be due to the relatively low susceptibility of malignant cells, the high body burden of tumour in patients, the inability to achieve satisfactory concentrations of the drugs in the centres of tumours, the eventual development of drug resistance by many tumours and the normal tissue toxicity induced by the agents[6].

This does not mean that good responses in assessable disease are not seen with single agents. Unfortunately, only patients achieving complete clinical remission are recognized to have any improvement in life expectancy, and this is a rare phenomenon. Clinical use of single agent chemotherapy established patterns of tumour response and identified the important dose limiting toxicity of individual agents.

The introduction of sequential courses of combinations of effective agents[79], chosen to achieve a clinically additive effect, without undue toxicity, has consistently altered the prognosis and resulted in long disease-free survival in a number of diseases. Unfortunately, it is the rarer testicular tumours, choriocarcinoma, Hodgkin's disease, Ewings sarcoma and acute lymphoblastic leukaemia of childhood that have shown maintained good responses to this type of treatment. The use of the word cure is difficult when patients have not been followed-up for many years but restoration of a normal life style and long survival are common in these diseases.

The patient with intractable pain is usually suffering from one of the disseminated solid tumours that does not enjoy a similar response to chemotherapy. Carcinomas of the breast, bronchus, gastrointestinal tract, kidney, bladder, prostate, cervix and ovary remain incurable in their metastatic forms. The patient's pain arises from only one facet of a disseminated incurable disease. Assessment of a wide varity of different combination chemotherapy regimes in these diseases has established the agents producing the best responses in measurable disease. These at the present moment vary from about 60% in breast cancer[80] to 0% in renal adenocarcinoma[81]. It should be noted that 'response' is defined in terms of objective changes in measurable disease and at present pain relief is not regarded as a meaningful response to anti-cancer drugs[6]. In addition no chemotherapy regime is without its toxicity and in a patient with symptoms from systemic disease there is always an important balance to be struck between the likely response, its duration and quality and the toxicity of the treatment. Unfortunately, even in very responsive diseases like breast cancer and small oat cell carcinoma of the bronchus the objective changes seen in different types of metastatic disease, soft tissue, parenchymal lung, liver, bone, CNS, vary enormously, with soft tissue disease usually the most sensitive while CNS metastases do not respond to combination chemotherapy.

A good example for those interested in pain management in multiple myeloma. This disseminated metastatic disease has bone pain as a very important prominent symptom. Local deposits of symptomatic disease respond to X-ray therapy but the disseminated nature of the disease has limited the use of this approach. The best combination chemotherapy regimes evolving from clinical studies do not produce cure but remissions of disease are relatively common and are associated with improved survival[82]. Objective bone healing can be observed in some of these responders[83,84] and this would be expected to be associated with relief of bone pain. Inevitably all responders relapse radiologically and symptomatically, usually in the face of continuing therapy[82].

At the present time it only appears justifiable to treat a patient in pain from metastatic malignant disease with combination chemotherapy if his problem comes from a type of disease which is consistently responsive, symptoms cannot be controlled by local X-ray therapy and his general condition is good enough to suggest that life expectancy can be measured in months rather than days or weeks.

Since systemic toxicity dictates the tolerance of the patient to chemotherapy two techniques continue to be used in an attempt to localize the treatment. Intra-arterial chemotherapy of localized troublesome deposits of malignant disease, e.g. recurrent head and neck cancer, pelvic tumours and liver metastases, has been explored for three decades.

Modern radiological techniques allow easy cannulation of afferent vascular supplies and the theoretical benefits of a highly localized concentrated chemotherapeutic treatment can be realized. The technique has, however, not achieved widespread acceptance. The problems preventing this have been the inevitable relapses with recurrence of symptoms in incurable patients and the devastating and unacceptable complications seen when local tissue tolerance is exceeded by the chemotherapy[85].

A more promising approach which has developed more recently has been to combine the chemotherapeutic agent with a carrier molecule that ensures a high uptake of the drug in the malignant disease so concentrating the effect and, hopefully, reducing systemic toxicity. The best example is Estra mustine, a combination of oestradiol-17ß and an alkylating agent. This has been developed for carcinoma of the prostate, a disease that can carry hormone receptors on the malignant cells (see the section on endocrinology). Early studies[86] have demonstrated subjective and objective responses in one third of patients with disease refractory to hormone therapy and X-ray therapy without significant systemic toxicity. These responses have included the unusual disappearance of blastic metastatic disease and significant remission of chronic pain.

CLINICAL PROBLEM AREAS

In spite of the advances discussed in the sections above there remain a number of clinical situations in which improved radiotherapeutic, chemotherapeutic, surgical and hormonal therapy have failed to make any significant impact and in which chronic pain is a major problem.

(1) Infiltration of the sciatic plexus or sacrum by invasive malignant disease – usually carcinoma of the cervix, rectum or bladder.
(2) Progressive infiltration after radiotherapy of the brachial plexus – usually in carcinoma of the breast or lung.
(3) Retro-peritoneal and coeliac axis malignant disease from gastro-intestinal, pancreatic or renal carcinoma.
(4) Rapidly developing liver metastases from any site.
(5) Progressive chest wall invasion – usually from carcinoma of the bronchus.

Patients with these types of metastatic disease represent very difficult management problems. Improved diagnostic techniques (cf. CAT scanning) may identify them at an earlier stage than previously and this in itself may allow at least some theoretical hope that earlier treatment may help to control the problem. It is, certainly, difficult to avoid attempting to treat patients with difficult symptoms from these complications but the wider availability of other pain controlling techniques and a clearer understanding of the limitations of present anti-cancer therapy would be of benefit to many patients.

HYPERTHERMIA

An unusual new approach to advanced malignant disease has emerged from the clinical observation that high temperatures can be associated with regression of metastatic disease. Using different techniques patients can be safely heated to 41–42 °C and this temperature maintained for 2–4 hours. Tumour regression and relief of pain have been recorded in advanced soft tissue sarcomas and gastrointestinal carcinomata[87]. More recently in less responsive disease, like breast cancer, the hyperthermia has been combined with chemotherapy and again good objective clinical responses and relief of pain are claimed[88]. The technique is strictly palliative and there are considerable risks associated with raising patients body temperatures but in experienced hands this can be achieved satisfactorily and it is certainly worthy of consideration in patients with severe symptoms from soft tissue sarcomas and gastrointestinal carcinomas if facilities are available locally.

CONCLUSION

For may patients cancer remains an incurable disease. Even for those with widespread symptomatic metastatic disease modern diagnostic aids discussed above and new approaches to therapy offer potential benefits to some patients. Careful patient selection and avoidance of the iatrogenic morbidity can hope to alleviate suffering during the terminal stages of disease. This unsatisfactory situation is likely to continue until methods of monitoring and controlling systemic solid tumours become widely available through clinical research.

References

1 Bourke R. S. (1976). Pain and its relief. *Int. J. Rad. Onc. Biol. Phys.*, **1**, 511
2 Cleland, W. P. (1972). The place of surgery in the treatment of carcinoma of the bron-

chus in modern radiotherapy. In Deeley, T. J. (ed.) *Modern Radiotherapy. Carcinoma of the Bronchus.* pp. 134–139 (London: Butterworths)

3 Mallams, J. T., Paulson, D. L., Collier, R. E. and Shaw, R. R. (1964). Pre-surgical irradiation in bronchogenic carcinoma superior sulcus type. *Radiology*, **82**, 1050

4 Lamesen, F., Rocmas, P. and Lustma, M. (1976). Pancoast syndrome and pulmonary sulcus tumours. *Rev. Franc. Mal. Resp.*, **11**, 883

5 Galasko, C. S. B. and Sylvester, B. S. (1978). Back pain in patients treated for malignant tumours. *Clin. Oncol.*, **4**, 273

6 Bonnadonna, G. and Molinari, R. (1976). Role and limits of anti-cancer drugs in the treatment of advanced cancer pain. In Bonica, J. J. and Ventafrida, V. (eds.), *Advances in Pain Research and Therapy.* Vol. 2. pp. 131–138 (New York: Raven Press)

7 Subramanian, G. and McAfee, J. G. (1971). New complex of ^{99m}Tc phosphate for skeletal imaging. *Radiology*, **99**, 192

8 Kirkman, S. and Henk, J. M. (1979). The value of bone scanning in the staging of breast cancer. *Clin. Radiol.*, **30**, 11

9 Silberstein, E. B. (1976). Causes of abnormalities reported in nuclear medicine testing. *J. Nucl. Med.*, **17**, 229

10 Galasko, C. S. B. (1978). Problems associated with the detection of skeletal metastases. *J. R. Soc. Med.*, **71**, 38

11 Roberts, J. G., Gravelle, I. H., Baum, M., Bugh, A. S., Leach, K. G. and Hughes, L. E. (1976). Evaluation of radiography and isotope scintigraphy for detecting skeletal metastases in breast cancer. *Lancet*, **1**, 237

12 Gillespie, P. J., Alexander, J. L. and Eddstyn, G. A. (1975). Changes in ^{87m}Sr. concentrations in skeletal metastases in patients responding to cyclical combination chemotherapy for advanced breast cancer. *J. Nucl. Med.*, **16**, 191

13 Larson, S. M. (1978). Mechanism of localization of Gallium 67 in tumours. *Semin. Nucl. Med.*, **3**, 193

14 Edward, C. L. and Hayes, R. L. (1970). Scanning malignant neoplasms with Gallium 67. *J. Am. Med. Assoc.*, **212**, 118

15 Krolikiewiez, H., Maruyama, Y., Deland, F. H., Beihn, R. M., Hafner, T. and Uhey, J. E. (1977). Localisation of Hodgkin's disease and lymphomas by Gallium-67 substraction scanning. *Onocolgy*, **34**, 179

16 Andrews, G. A., Hubner, K. F. and Greenlow, W. (1978). Ga^{67} citrate imaging in malignant lymphoma. Final report of a co-operative group. *J. Nucl. Med.*, **19**, 1013

17 Johnson, G. S. (1977). Gallium 67 citrate imaging in Hodgkin's disease. Final report of co-operative group. *J. Nucl. Med.*, **18**, 692

18 Tyrrell, C. J., Cosgrove, D. O., McCready, V. R. and Peckham, M. J. (1977). The role of ultrasound in the assessment and treatment of abdominal metastases from testicular tumours. *Clin. Radiol.*, **28**, 475

19 Wright, C. H., Mankead, M. F. and Rosenthal, S. J. (1979). Grey scale ultrasound characteristics of carcinoma of the pancreas. *Br. J. Radiol.*, **52**, 281

20 Miere, H. B. and Kreel, L. (1978). Computed tomography and ultrasound, a comparison. *Practitioner*, **220**, 593

21 Miere, H. B. (1979). Diagnostic ultrasound. *Br. J. Radiol.*, **52**, 685

22 Kreel, L. (1978). Computed axial tomography in the diagnosis and treatment of malignancy. *Cancer Treatment Rev.*, **5**, 117

23 Kreel, L. (1976). The EMI whole body scanner in the demonstration of lymph node enlargement. *Clin. Radiol.*, **27**, 421

24 Stephens, D. H., Sheady, P. F., Hattery, R. R. and Williamson, B. (1977). Diagnosis and evaluation of retro-peritoneal tumours by computed tomography. *Am. J. Roent.*, **129**, 395

25 Husband, J. E. and Kreel, L. (1978). Computerised tomography in the demonstration of lymph node enlargement. *J. R. Soc. Med.,* **71,** 35

26 Bagshawe, K. (1975). *Medical Oncology.* Chap. 13, p. 245. (Oxford: Blackwell Scientific Publications)

27 Sugarbaker, P. H., Zamcheck, N. and Moore, F. D. (1976). Assessment of serial carcinoembryonic antigen (CEA) assays in postoperative detection of recurrent colon carcinoma. *Cancer,* **38,** 2310

28 Grigor, K. M., Detrie, S. I., Kohn, J. and Neville, A. M. (1977). Serial α-foetoprotein levels in 153 male patients with germ cell tumours. *Br. J. Cancer.,* **35,** 52

29 Lokich, J. J., Zamchek, M. and Lowenstein, M. (1978). Sequential carcinoembryonic antigen levels in the therapy of metastatic breast cancer. *Ann. Intern. Med.,* **89,** 902

30 Jackson, S. M. (1978). In Swerdlow, M. (ed.). *Relief of Intractable Pain.* pp. 285–317. 2nd edn. (Amsterdam: Excepta Medica)

31 Boland, J., Glicksman, A. and Vargha, A. O. (1969). Single dose radiation therapy in the palliation of metastatic disease. *Radiology,* **93,** 1181

32 Jensen, N. H. and Roesdam, K. (1976). Single dose irradiation of bone metastases. *Acta Radiol. Ther. Phys. Biol.,* **15,** 337

33 Allen, K. L., Johnson, T. W. and Hibbs, G. G. (1976). Effective bone palliation as related to various treatment regimens. *Cancer,* **37,** 984

34 Penn, C. R. H. (1976). Single dose and fractionated palliative irradiation for osseous metastases. *Clin. Radiol.,* **27,** 405

35 Hendrickson, F. R. and Sheinkop, M. B. (1975). Management of osseous metastases. *Semin. Oncol.,* **2,** 4

36 Galasko, C. S. B., Bush, H. and Sutton, M. (1980). In Halnan, K. E. (ed.). *Bone Synovium and Cartilage in Treatment of Cancer.* (In press)

37 Rubin, P. and Scarantino, C. W. (1978). The bone marrow organ; the critical structure in radiation–drug interaction. *Int. J. Radiat. Oncol. Biol. Phys.,* **4,** 3

38 Fitzpatrick, P. J. and Rider, W. D. (1976). Half body radiotherapy. *Int. J. Radiat. Oncol. Biol. Phys.,* **1,** 197

39 Rowland, C. G. (1979). Single fraction half body radiation therapy. *Clin. Radiol.,* **30,** 1

40 Dawes, P. J. D. K. (1979). Acute pulmonary distress following high dose irradiation of the upper half of the body. *Br. J. Radiol.,* **52,** 876

41 Galasko, C. S. B. (1976). Mechanism of bone destruction in the development of skeletal metastases. *Nature (London),* **263,** 507

42 Galasko, C. S. B. and Bennett, A. (1976). Relationship of bone destruction in skeletal metastases to tumours containing high concentrations of prostaglandin like material. *Nature (London),* **263,** 508

43 Bonarigo, B. C. and Rubin, P. (1967). The non-union of pathologic fracture after radiation therapy. *Radiology,* **88,** 889

44 Douglas, H. O., Shukla, S. K. and Mindell, E. (1976). Treatment of pathological fractures of long bones excluding those due to breast cancer. *J. Bone Jt. Surg. Ser. A.,* **58,** 1055

45 Ricci, S. B. (1979). Radiation therapy. In Bonica, J. J. and Ventrafridda, V. (eds.). *Advances in Pain Research and Therapy.* Vol. 2, pp. 167–174 (New York: Raven Press)

46 Johnson, D. and Haynie, T. P. (1977). [32]P for intractable pain in cancer of the prostate. *Urology,* **2,** 137

47 Maxfield, J. R., Maxfield, J. G. S. and Maxfield, W. S. (1958). The use of radio-active phosphorus and testosterone in metastatic bone lesions from breast and prostate. *S. Med. J.,* **51,** 320

48 Donati, R. M., Ellis, H. and Gallagher, M. I. (1966). Testosterone potentiated ^{32}P therapy in prostatic cancer. *Cancer,* **19,** 1088

49 Klinger, L. (1974). Polyphosphate bone scans, ^{32}phosphorus and adenocarcinoma of the thyroid. *J. Nucl. Med.*, **15**, 1037

50 Firusion, N., Mevin, P. and Schmidt, C. G. (1976). Results of ^{89}Sr therapy in patients with cancer of the prostate and incurable pain from bone metastases. *J. Urol.*, **116**, 764

51 Harrington, K. D., Sim, F., Johnson, J., Dick, H. and Gristina, A. G. (1976). Trimethylmethacrylate as an adjunct in internal fixation of pathological fractures. *J. Bone Jt. Surg.*, **58**, 1047

52 McAusland, W. R. and Wyman, E. T. (1970). Management of metastatic pathological fractures. *Clin. Orth.*, **73**, 39

53 Parrish, F. F. and Murray, J. A. (1970). Treatment of metastatic bone disease. *J. Bone Jt. Surg.*, **52**, 65

54 Douglas, H. D., Shukla, S. K. and Mindell, E. (1974). Treatment of pathological fractures of long bones excluding those due to breast cancer. *J. Bone Jt. Surg.*, **58**, 1055

55 Fidler, M. (1973). Prophylactic internal fixation of secondary neoplastic deposits in long bones. *Br. Med. J.*, **1**, 341

56 Francis, W. (1970). The role of amputation in the treatment of metastatic bone cancer. *Clin. Orth.*, **73**, 61

57 McGuire, W. L., Carbone, P. P. and Volmer E. (1975). *Oestrogen Receptors in Human Breast Cancer.* (Amsterdam: North Holland)

58 Laing, L., Calman, K. C., Smith, M. G., Smith, D. C. and Leake, R. E. (1977). Nuclear oestrogen receptors in prediction of response to therapy of breast cancer. *Lancet*, **2**, 168

59 King, R. J. B. and Roberts, M. (1979). In King, R. (ed.). *Steroid Receptor Assays in Human Breast Tumours.* Chap. 1, p. 1–6. (Cardiff: Alpha and Omega Publishing)

60 Barnes, D. M., Ribeiro, G. G. and Skinner, L. G. (1979). In King, R. (ed.). *Steroid Receptor Assays in Human Breast Tumours.* Chap. 3, pp. 16–32. (Cardiff: Alpha and Omega Publishing)

61 Statement by the British Breast Group and colleagues. (1980). Steroid receptor assays in human breast cancer. *Lancet*, **1**, 298

62 Barnes, D. M., Skinner, L. G. and Ribeiro, G. G. (1979). Triple hormone receptor assay. A more accurate predictive tool for the treatment of advanced breast cancer. *Br. J. Cancer*, **40**, 862

63 Menon, M., Tavarins, C. E., McLoughlin, M. G. and Walsh, P. C. (1978). Androgen receptors in tumour prostatic tissue; a review. *Cancer Treatment Rep.*, **61**, 265

64 Nijs, M., Brassino, C. and Cowne, A. (1979). Steroid receptors in human prostate cancer. *Cancer Treatment Rep.*, **63**, 1194

65 Ekman, P. (1979). Steroid receptor assay in human prostatic carcinoma for prediction of tumour response to endocrine therapy. *Cancer treatment Rep.*, **63**, 1188

66 Gustaffson, J., Stockowsk, M., Zetterberg, A., Povselte, A. and Hogberg, B. (1978). Correlation between clinical response to hormone therapy and steroid receptor content in prostatic cancer. *Cancer Res.*, **38**, 4345

67 Ferguson, J. D. and Hendrey, W. F. (1971). Pituitary irradiation in advanced carcinoma of the prostate. *Br. J. Urol.*, **43**, 514

68 Silverberg, G. D. (1977). Hypophysectomy in the treatment of disseminated prostate carcinoma. *Cancer*, **39**, 1727

69 Levin, A. B., Benson C. C., Katz, J. and Nilson, J. (1978). Clinical hypophysectomy for relief of bone pain in carcinoma of the prostate. *J. Urol.*, **119**, 517

70 Gye, R. S., Stanworth, P. A., Stewart, J. A. and Adams, C. B. T. (1979). Cryohypophysectomy for bone pain of metastatic breast carcinoma. *Pain*, **6**, 201

71 Harrold, B. P., Cotes, J. E. and James, J. A. (1968). Treatment of advanced breast cancer by transphenoidal hypophysectomy. *Br. J. Cancer.*, **22**, 19

72 Roberts, M. M. (1970). A comparison of transphenoidal hypophysectomy and Yttrium 90 implant and adrenalectomy. In Joslin, C. and Gleave, E. M. (eds.). *The Clinical Management of Advanced Breast Cancer.* p. 54. (Cardiff: Alpha and Omega Press)

73 Morrell, H., Alves, A. M., Winternitz, W. W. and Maddy, J. (1970). A clinicopathological analysis of cryohypophysectomy in patients with advanced cancer. *Cancer*, **25**, 1050

74 LaRossa, J. T., Strong, M. S. and Melby, J. C. (1978). Endocrinologically incomplete transethmoidal transphenoidal hypophysectomy with relief of bone pain in breast cancer. *N. Engl. J. Med.*, **298**, 1332

75 Baron, D. M., Gurlins, K. J. and Radley-Smith, E. J. (1958). The effect of hypophysectomy in advanced carcinoma of the breast. *Br. J. Surg.*, **45**, 593

76 Moricca, J. (1976). Neuro adenolysis for diffuse unbearable cancer pain. In Bonica, J. J. and Albe-Fessard, D. (eds.). *Advances in Pain Research and Therapy.* Vol. 1, pp. 863–866. (New York: Raven Press)

77 Lipton, S., Miles, J., Williams, N. and Bark Jones, M. (1978). Pituitary injection of alcohol for widespread cancer pain. *Pain*, **5**, 73–82

78 Tindall, G. T., Nixon, D. W., Christy, J. H. and Neill J. D. (1977). Pain relief in metastatic carcinoma other than breast and prostate gland following transphenoidal hypophysectomy. *J. Neursurg.*, **47**, 659

79 Devita, V. T. and Shein, P. S. (1973). Use of drugs in combination for the treatment of cancer. *N. Engl. J. Med.*, **288**, 998

80 Canellos, G. P., Devita, V. T., Gold, G. L., Chasmer, E. A., Schein, P. S. and Young, R. C. (1974). Cyclical combination chemotherapy for advanced breast carcinoma. *Br. Med. J.*, **1**, 218

81 Bodey, G. P. (1979). Current status of chemotherapy in metastatic renal carcinoma. In Johnson, D. E. and Samuels, M. L. (eds.). *Cancer of the Genito-urinary Tract.* (New York: Raven Press)

82 Alexanian, R., Salmon, S. E., Bonnet, J., Gehan, E., Hant, A. and Weik, J. (1977). Combination therapy for multiple myeloma. *Cancer*, **40**, 2765

83 Dawson, W. B. (1968). Sclerotic repair of myelomatous bone defects following chemotherapy. *Clin. Radiol.*, **19**, 323

84 Rodriquez, L. H., Finklestein, B., Schullemberger, C. C., Alexanian, R. (1972). Bone healing in multiple myeloma with melphalan chemotherapy. *Ann. Intern. Med.*, **76**, 551

85 Nevin, J. E., Melnick, I., Baggerly, J. T., Hoffman, A., Landes, R. and Easley, C. (1973). The continuous arterial infusion of 5FU as a therapeutic adjuvant in the treatment of advanced carcinoma of the bladder and prostate. *Cancer*, **31**, 138

86 Murphy, G. P. (1979). *Chemotherapeutic treatment on a National Randomized Trial Basis by the National Prostatic Cancer Project.* In Johnson, D. E. and Samuels, M. L. (eds.). *Cancer of the Genito-urinary Tract.* p. 249. (New York: Raven Press)

87 Pettigrew, R. J., Galt, J. M., Ludgate, C. M. and Smith A. N. (1974). Clinical effects of whole body hyperthermia in advanced malignancy. *Br. Med. J.*, **4**, 679

88 Moricca, G., Cavaliere, R., Lopez, M. and Carvto, A. (1979). Combined whole body hyperthermia and chemotherapy in the treatment of advanced cancer with diffuse pain. In Bonica, J. J. and Ventafridda, V. (eds.). *Advances in Pain Research and Therapy.* Vol. 2, pp. 195–210 (New York: Raven Press)

9

Current views on
pain relief and terminal care

Cicely Saunders

> *'The last act crowns the play', (Francis Quarles)*

Sadly, the terminal stage could be defined as beginning at the moment when a clinician says, 'There is nothing more to be done' and begins to withdraw from contact with the patient. To say this, as Smithers has pointed out, 'is inexcusable and seldom if ever true'[1]. Patients and their families are well aware when this happens and their feelings of isolation add to the total experience of pain.

The use of the word terminal has also tended to obscure the fact that it does not always refer to an irreversible state. Terminal care is a facet of oncology (and of other disciplines also), being concerned with the control of symptoms of the disease process once that has become uncontrollable.

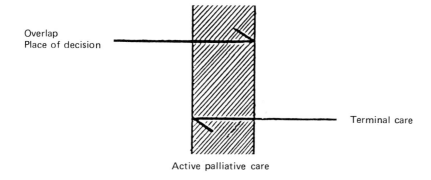

Overlap
Place of decision

Terminal care

Active palliative care

Figure 1 The initiation of terminal care

The effective relief of pain and other symptoms by terminal care may accompany or revive the prospect of further acute palliative care. No patient should become locked in what may become for him the wrong therapeutic system. The aims of the two are not mutually exclusive and there is a considerable area of overlap, as shown in Figure 1. When competent control of symptoms accompanies palliative therapy, it is often less difficult for the clinician to recognize the moment when the latter becomes irrelevant and should be withdrawn.

INCIDENCE

Table 1 summarizes reports from four studies concerning the incidence of unrelieved terminal pain. Except for Woodbine, they refer to retrospective evidence. Turnbull's figures come from his perusal of hospital and pain relief clinic notes and the others from the memories of the surviving spouses. They suggest that it is not unduly pessimistic to estimate that about one third of all patients who died of malignant disease are remembered later by those in close contact with them as having had poor pain relief. If we compare this figure with the Registrar General's total of 126 788 deaths from cancer in 1978 we must estimate that over 42 000 people during that year are likely to have had a substantial amount of unrelieved pain during their terminal illness.

Table 1 Incidence of unrelieved terminal pain

Date reported	Author	Number of patients	Incidence of unrelieved pain
1954	Turnbull	100	38% ('intractable')
1959	Aitken and Swan	200	20% ('unrelieved') 18% ('relieved to some extent' or 'at the end')
1977	Woodbine	97	34% Home 34% Hospital ('moderate or severe pain during previous 24 hours')
1978	Parkes	276	28% Home 20% Hospital 8% Hospice ('severe pain mostly unrelieved')

Many of these patients will not have endured prolonged pain. Pain may be a feature early in recurrent disease for some patients but the terminal period itself is likely to be comparatively short. Few patients with terminal malignant disease receive the Attendance Allowance because most of them do not fulfil the qualifying 6 months of attendance from another person before their death. Parkes' study from which Figure 2 is taken was carried out during 1967–72. It showed that among 276 married patients under the age of 65 who died of cancer in two London boroughs, 49 were still under active treatment at the time of death and that while the length of time after the end of such treatment varied greatly, the median length of stay for terminal care was 9 weeks. Parkes divided these patients into *home based*, including in this group all who died within a week of a final hospital admission, *hospital based* and *St. Christopher's based*. The amount of pre-terminal pain and terminal pain reported by their next of kin afterwards[2] is shown in Figure 2. This study is being repeated 10 years later as part of the evaluation of the work of the Hospice.

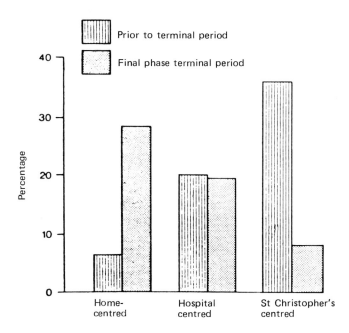

Figure 2 Proportions of patients with severe and mostly continuous pain (after Parkes)

Although retrospective studies based on family memories are likely to be biased by confused and confusing feelings such as guilt at allowing a patient to go to hospital, rationalization at not bringing him home and the projection of the angry feelings so common in bereavement, these figures are substantiated by Woodbine's observations. He interviewed 97 patients identified by their doctors for whom no further curative treatment was appropriate, 63 at home and 34 in hospital. 34% of both groups reported moderate or severe pain in the 24 hours prior to interview, despite a variety of drugs. He comments that the medication written up only rarely included the narcotic analgesics and that of the 29 patients with pain only four 'received strong pain drugs on the day of interview'[3].

Another disturbing paper has shown how much pain goes unrecognized in a general teaching hospital where 'nurses accept the presence of unrelieved pain in patients too readily, as indicated by the practice of confining enquiry about pain to drug rounds and by ignoring non-verbal communication[4].

Table 2 shows that for the past 6 years only 1% of patients at St. Christopher's have had continuing pain problems. These figures are based on the assessment of pain control made by a research nurse and a doctor not involved with the care given on the wards from the twice daily nursing notes and clinician's reports.

Table 2 Pain in patients with malignant disease from 1972 to 1977

Year	Number of patients	Pain difficult to control (no of cases)
1972	480	7
1973	555	7
1974	534	7
1975	595	5
1976	607	6
1977	591	2
Total	3362	34 (1%)

Mount reports a series of studies which showed that oral morphine may be tolerated in approximately 85–90% of patients and that as high a proportion as 95% will attain excellent pain control[5]. An earlier paper showed that the Brompton mixture 'was strikingly more effective than the traditional methods of managing cancer pain'[6].

In 1971, Evans reported on the first five years of a pain clinic in Toronto and stated that he found intractable pain in only 0.5% of all the cancer patients attending that hospital[7]. This is a different population from the St. Christopher's patients, who all have advanced disease and the majority of whom are referred by doctors who have found their symptoms difficult to control. These reports and others show that the skill to change the figures shown in Table 1 already exists and should be made available to every patient with terminal pain.

THE NATURE OF TERMINAL PAIN

Although the terminal period of persistent malignant disease is often brief compared with some forms of chronic disease, its course (and its treatment) frequently delivers a series of blows, each destroying some part of the patient's capacity for normal and independent living. One is constantly amazed at the endurance and resilience shown by the great majority and at the rarity of severe reaction depressions. Pain can blot out the world, cut off all true communication and perpetually renew a vicious circle of pain, fear, tension and further pain. It is no exaggeration to term a patient's suffering as 'total pain' and it may help to divide it into physical, emotional, social and spiritual components in order to assess, understand and treat these people and their feelings better. The pain which causes an animal to remain motionless while an injured part heals is a total 'feeling state'. Wall, in his recent John Bonica lecture, suggests that pain is better classified as a need state than as a sensation, serving more to promote healing than to avoid injury[8]. Terminal pain is certainly a need state but it rarely promotes healing and has no such built in meaning for those who suffer it. Rather it traps the patient in a situation for which there is no reassuring explanation and to which there is no foreseeable end. This is a radically different pain from the post-operative pain which has been researched by many workers from Beecher onwards[9] and which forms a large part of teaching hospital experience.

Patients referred to the hospice for inpatient care or out-patient support are those with problems previously found difficult to solve. It is therefore not surprising that in 1978 over 77% of them should have presented with pain as a major problem and that nearly all required narcotic drugs before death or discharge. During 1976 an assessment was made of the social problems reported on admission and in 75.5% of the patients these had helped to precipitate admission. It is when problems add up to a total pain situation that the family is overwhelmed and home care breaks down.

219

ASSESSMENT AND ANALYSIS

It is revealing to find how many patients with terminal disease are surprised to find a doctor who will listen to the story of their pain. As we listen to each one and to his family we are assessing the nature of the pain on the physical level, identifying its nature, sites and possible causes, but also analysing its implications for this individual, in the light of his own family, background and culture, past experience and present anxieties.

If we are to ensure continuity of care for him and his family we must learn all we can of a patient's history. Care for such a person calls for good liaison between hospital departments and between them and the new unit or the family doctor. The last is often poor. Letters and reports are delayed, nothing of what has been said to the patient or the family is passed on and they are left completely in the dark as to what to expect[10]. The doctor in the new unit may have to be most importunate in demanding full reports from doctors, social workers and ward nurses if he is to begin on the solid ground of adequate past records.

It is the custom in St. Christopher's to see the family while the patient is being settled into the ward. If he is not in acute pain and does not need immediate attention this is to be preferred. It is also important to discover from the family what has been happening at home and to gain some idea of the speed of the changes in the patient's physical state. Patients are often unrealistic about their own mobility and sleep at night and may forget dates and details without being in any way confused. As we try to find out from the family in what terms the patient is talking about his illness, we may learn as much about their attitude as about his and be able to make some assessment of the fears and problems of all concerned. This serves to review the past in their terms and to give them the assurance that all future care will involve them and their needs.

The answer given by a patient to the question 'Tell me about your illness (or your pain)', is most revealing. He describes the symptoms which are troubling him most and conveys a great deal about his insight. People often have greater knowledge than those around them are able or willing to recognize and it is not always the obvious physical problems that call for the most urgent attention. His question about the symptoms and his physical examination enable the doctor to diagnose and plan treatment for the terminal pain as a kind of disease in itself and are often therapeutic especially when time is taken for some kind of explanation of what has been found and what will be done to help. Pain and other symptoms are not always directly due to the malignant process and general medicine is no more to be neglected here than in any other branch of medical practice; much distress can be relieved without the use of analgesics. The patient's general condition, independence and mobility may be improved by an adequate plan of symptomatic treatment and by comparatively simple measures. For example haemorrhoids, bad teeth and dyspepsia still give pain when the sufferer is terminally ill and respond to the usual treatments. Whatever confidence he has had in his previous doctors, a fresh assessment and a determined approach to symptom control begin to restore a person's importance as an individual of value. Many have had this much undermined by all that has happened. At this stage, nurses of every rank and the whole ward team should be involved. The physiotherapist, the occupational or diversional therapist, the social worker and the chaplain may have much to contribute. The patient now knows not only that some kind of base line concerning his physical state has been established but also that he has been seen as a particular person who is part of a unique family. Isolation and anonymity are likely to have been his worst suffering and to have added greatly to his physical distress.

REFERRAL TO OTHER DISCIPLINES

Judgements concerning referral to other disciplines must be made as soon as possible for these patients have little time. Every unit or team specializing in terminal care must develop its own multi-disciplinary links and keep its communication system in good order. Each has its own strengths and weaknesses and one needs to be realistic and effective in exploiting the one and circumventing the other.

The radiotherapy and oncology departments and the pain relief clinic are likely to be called on most often, although the skill of any of the specialities of the general hospital may be needed. Each hospice unit will discover those who are most interested in such referrals. Most patients are also glad when their previous specialist is called in again or when he makes a follow up visit even if this is mainly social in nature.

Palliative radiotherapy may be most effective even now (for the relief of pain, provided it is applied skilfully. Radiotherapy may also be considered for the relief of haemoptysis, haematuria or vaginal bleeding, all very disturbing to the patient and the family. It may be used to control fungation and discharge and to control cough and dyspnoea by treating either the primary tumour or mediastinal and other lymph nodes[11].

Regular rounds with a radiotherapist and oncologist are an essential for a hospice unit, not only to discuss the patients selected by the terminal care team but also to review others who could benefit. Such rounds have taken place quarterly over the past years at St. Christopher's Hospice. Initially, they identified some 5% of the total patient population as still likely to benefit. Such patients, now recognized by the hospice team themselves, are frequently discussed by telephone with the radiotherapist and this liaison is as straightforward as that of a unit which is part of a general hospital. A group of patients with advanced breast cancer come to a regular joint out-patient clinic. Such shared care will give an unexpected extra lease of life to the few, help in pain relief for a substantial minority and keep the options open for the unexpected reversal of the disease process for all.

A similar exercise has recently been carried out to reassess the possibilities of a closer link with a pain relief clinic. During the past year a series of rounds which reviewed all patients in 62 beds were carried out. As the hospice has a median stay of 11–12 days, many patients were too ill to be considered but of the remainder some 10% were thought likely to benefit from the clinic's treatments. Twenty-six procedures were carried out in the hospice on 12 patients with 15 separate pains, eight of whom had good, lasting relief. In addition to these patients, six others were assessed but not treated and a further 25 patients were discussed. Some of this group were presented for discussion, while a few (5–10 only) were considered seriously for assessment but were felt to be either too ill for treatment or too likely to suffer undesirable side effects.

At another hospice a daily visit by the pain clinic anaesthetist has resulted in various techniques being used for 22.7% of the patients admitted, including cervical subdural phenol, epidural/intrathecal phenol, coeliac plexus block and pituitary alcohol injections[12].

These joint rounds have been of benefit to a substantial number of patients and have educated the doctors on both sides. It is to be hoped that with the proliferation of pain relief clinics and hospice teams it will become part of the accepted traditions of both. For some patients one or other of the disciplines will give the better treatment, others will need a combination of skills. In areas where there is no hospice, the pain clinic will support those terminally ill patients referred to it for pain control.

Transcutaneous stimulators have not so far had great success in the Hospice; we have no personal experience with hypnosis and acupuncture, more from their non-availability than from lack of interest. Others may wish to explore these and other possibilities for their dying patients.

So long as they are part of a general medical approach and no patient fails to have access to other therapies he may need and so long as their results are adequately monitored and evaluated one could not question their use, remembering how great a part interest and enthusiasm play in giving relief to these patients.

ON THE USE OF ANALGESICS FOR TERMINAL PAIN

While there is no need to resort automatically to strong analgesics when a patient approaches the terminal stages of his illness, pain must certainly be relieved as soon as it becomes a matter for complaint. We may have to elicit such complaint, for these patients often underestimate our interest in their pain or the possibility of relief; they do not like to bother us, even when pain is severe[4]. They rarely seek help without good cause. Adequate relief must be given from the beginning of the patient's down-hill course, for he should become accustomed to expect freedom from discomfort rather than its constant presence. The impact of pain is greatly influenced by past experience of pain and in turn it builds the expectation of future pain. If fear is aroused it will immediately enhance pain by tension. Such tension underlines its threat and once it has become established, pain is likely to need larger doses for its relief. The dramatic ease that may be given by an injection as a drug enters the blood stream naturally enhances any tendency to rely upon drugs. Crises that may call for injections should be anticipated and prevented wherever possible.

Mild terminal pain

The relief of mild terminal pain can usually be achieved with weak analgesics. This pain may not change in character and continue to respond to them throughout an entire illness. Even when more severe pain has supervened it is often surprising how useful such drugs remain. A well-tried remedy in which a patient has built up confidence over the months may be used as a standby to supplement more powerful medication, nor should we hesitate to allow our patients to use a favourite proprietory mixture in this way so long as we know what it contains.

In the view of many hospice doctors aspirin and to a lesser extent paracetamol are still the most useful remedies for mild pain in terminal illness. The dangers of aspirin in this situation are not great in propor-tion to the number of patients who will benefit and they are acceptable.

Gastric upset is more common but can usually be avoided by a sensible routine for taking medication, by trying different presentations of this valuable and versatile drug and by the use of antacids. It is important to discover a patient's preferences and idiosyncrasies.

Many drugs may be effective at this stage. In spite of its unimpressive performance in clinical trials and recent evidence of its potential dangers with overdose, dextropropoxyphene with or without paracetamol or aspirin (as Distalgesic, Doloxene or Darvon) continues to be widely used. At St. Christopher's we give 12–14 tablets in 24 hours with effect and safety.

Enthusiasm, careful instruction and the doctor's own confidence often do more to relieve terminal pain than any drugs. We need to employ competent therapy but it is because enthusiastic interest is so often denied to the patient with terminal cancer that his pain becomes so fraught with misery. The use of various adjuvant drugs should be considered at this stage and reviewed later if pain escalates. These will include the non-steroidal anti-inflammatory drugs for bone pain, steroids for raised intra-cranial pressure and for oedema causing nerve compression or around lymph node masses, treatment for infections, for bladder or bowel distension or disturbances, excoriated skin from incontinence and decubitus. Any painful pathology should be considered and dealt with specifically where possible.

The use of mild analgesics may be combined with small doses of one or more of the psychotropic drugs. Drugs of the phenothiazine group are not always used with the discrimination they warrant. They may remove nausea, ease anxiety, help to control confusion and calm restlessness. They also enhance the effect of analgesics. While we await more definitive studies we rely mainly on clinical experience in making our choice between them. An effective antiemetic with little sedative effect, such as prochlorperazine (Stemetil, Compazine) may be added to any analgesic at this stage. At the hospice it is prescribed for most patients when morphine is introduced but may be withdrawn after a few days if nausea is no problem. There is some evidence that trifluoperazine (Stelazine) may help to focus attention in those who for various organic reasons are confused. Chlorpromazine (Largactil, Thorazine) is still the best all-purpose drug in this group and is frequently used for sedation at night and for confusion with restlessness. This will be commonly prescribed in a starting dose of 10–12.5 mg t.d.s. or 4-hourly. A syrup preparation is often more easily swallowed and is also less likely to be refused by the suspicious and paranoid who are sometimes adept at removing their pills after the nurse with the drug round has disappeared.

The benzodiazepines have virtually replaced the barbiturates for the treatment of anxiety and tension in terminal illness. Diazepam may be a valuable addition and has also helped many relatives of dying patients to keep going so long as the dose prescribed was not too high. Used specifically for painful muscle spasm it is probably more satisfactory than baclofen, which can make some patients distressingly floppy.

The place of the tricyclic antidepressants in the field of pain control has not yet been elucidated and the evidence so far is nearly all anecdotal. Both patients and family members may occasionally need them for frank depression. Sorrow must be distinguished from this for it is appropriate and needs a listener rather than drugs, while symptom control will usually relieve mild depression. The longer the terminal phase lasts the higher the percentage of patients for whom these drugs are prescribed.

Pain rarely exists alone in these patients and excellence in its control demands excellence in the control of all other symptoms as well. Full reviews, summarizing their causes and suggestions for their rational treatment are given by Baines[13, 14] and Mount[15]. Constipation requires special mention since it is so common and can be so distressing that it needs to be considered and prevented wherever possible. The combined effect of loss of appetite and poor intake, a degree of dehydration, inactivity and narcotic and other therapy almost invariably lead to poor bowel motility. Very sick patients rarely tolerate bran or maintain a sufficient fluid intake to combine with the bulk-forming laxatives. A combination of a stool softener with a bowel stimulant such as Dorbanex Medo or Forte is usually effective but this will be a constant challenge to the nursing staff.

Dehydration rarely needs vigorous correction in the terminal weeks. Patients receiving narcotics seldom complain of thirst for it is relieved by narcotics together with other physical distress and patients do not welcome the discomfort of an intravenous drip. Small, frequent drinks, especially those offered by the family, ice with various flavours to suck and meticulous mouth care are far more comforting and effective.

Most of these measures should have been considered while the patient is still having active palliative treatment. Relief, like pain, is self-perpetuating. The early, imaginative and confident use of all these measures will add to the number of patients dying of malignant disease who never need strong analgesics.

Moderate terminal pain

Moderate pain may be relieved by one of a number of analgesics but the well tried codein has not been surpassed and serves as a standard. There are a number of drugs that appear to be equianalgesic in studies but vary in their clinical effectiveness. Dihydrocodeine will help one patient and render another intractably constipated. Dipipanone Co (Diconal) is more powerful. It keeps some patients fully mobile and has been reported as of especial value among patients with multiple myelomatosis receiving chemotherapy[16]. Other patients are rendered so drowsy and lethargic (possibly by the amount of cyclizine in each tablet) that they cannot take them at all. There is no evidence that dipipanone is any more nauseating than other analgesics but it is not obtainable alone. This is unfortunate since as a general rule mixed preparations are to be avoided and it is better to discover a patient's own best combination of drugs.

In our view there is little place for the use of pentazocine or pethidine in terminal care. Neither is a potent oral analgesic and both are comparatively short-acting. Pentazocine has the additional drawback of causing an unacceptably high incidence of psychotomimetic side effects. Dextromoramide is more potent but relatively short-acting and a considerable number of patients are admitted to St. Christopher's taking this drug 2 or even 1-hourly. It is useful, however, as a cover for a painful episode when given as a supplement to other regular medication. Papaveretum and opium are frequently combined with aspirin and are given for moderate pain, often over long periods, in radiotherapy departments and some of the hospices.

Morphine and diamorphine may be used to control moderate pain in small doses (such as 5–10 mg oral morphine). There is no constant pattern of dose increase and patients are often maintained on the same dose for weeks or months. Nor is there any problem in reducing the dose or withdrawing the narcotic altogether if pain control is achieved by other means.

Analgesics may need to be used as suppositories in home care. In our hands morphine by this route has not been as effective as oxycodone pectinate, (Proladone). Used at 8 or sometimes 6-hourly intervals it may make home care a possibility for patients with severe pain who can take nothing by mouth. Chlorpromazine and prochlorperazine suppositories should be added for patients with nausea and/or vomiting and may be considered if a patient's injection sites become painful.

Severe terminal pain

Misconceptions concerning the use of the strong analgesics continue to deny patients the relief that they should have. Fear of producing toler-

226

ance and psychological dependence is prevalent. Repeated escalations of dose are expected and a time when nothing is effective is quite erroneously considered to be inevitable. It is thought that there is no middle road between a patient in pain and one heavily sedated and because no proper standard of pain relief with unaffected sensorium exists in the clinician's mind he accepts these alternatives. One of the best known writers on pain considers that there is an endemic inadequacy in pain control[17] and our experience would certainly endorse this view.

Although new understanding of pain mechanisms and analgesic action may alter our approach and give us new tools during the next decade, patients need relief now and should expect any doctor to know how to provide it. No foreseeable number of hospices or pain clinics is going to reach the great majority of the terminally ill who are at present suffering pain and other physical distress, nor would it be right that such units or teams should undertake the care of all these patients as an exclusive speciality. Skill and confidence in handling analgesics and their adjuvants must become part of general medical education and whoever treats these patients must know when to begin with narcotic drugs, what routine to establish and what other medications to combine with them.

WHEN TO BEGIN

When terminal pain escapes control or when the patient finds he has to swallow more than two pills to obtain relief it is time for the smaller dose of a stronger drug. Vigorous effort must be made again to identify the cause of the increased pain, but there is no need to deny a patient relief of severe pain while its detailed aetiology is investigated. If a specific means of treating the pain is found, there need be no problem in withdrawing narcotic drugs as patients do not ask for them once their pain is relieved by other means. Physical signs of withdrawal are rare and if they occur will be avoided by reducing the dose over several days.

ROUTINE FOR PAIN PREVENTION

The typical pain of terminal cancer is constant in character, although it may have exacerbations such as on movement. Constant pain calls for constant control, not a desperate switchback between bouts of pain and periods of somnolent relief. Pain itself is the strongest antagonist to the drugs given to suppress it and it is of cardinal importance that neither its presence nor its threat should act against relief. If a patient has to ask for his analgesic he will be reminded each time of his dependence on the drug and on the person who gives it to him. If it is given regularly with a slightly relaxed schedule so that no one is obsessively clockwatching and at a dose that covers the extra period of relief that may be required should a dose be delayed, then pain can be forgotten and the self perpetuating spiral of misery and dependence is not initiated. Continual expectation of the recurrence of pain with p.r.n. narcotic orders or even with 'self demand' analgesia is the route to iatrogenically induced dependence.

Vere has shown[20] how the regular giving of oral narcotics prevents pain breakthrough by keeping the blood level continuously in the patient's own effective zone and below the level of toxicity. Oral doses facilitate this by yielding a more rounded peak than intravenous administration. Doses shuld be regularly spaced, including a night dose for most patients, who will prefer being woken for a dose rather than by pain some time later. "Unfortunately some strange parsimony seems to make doctors prescribe opiates 'as required', and an even stranger parsimony seems to prevent them being given even when they are required. The only way to avoid both problems is never to use 'as required' prescriptions in this context[20]."

As Vere points out and as many years of experience have shown, tolerance is not a clinical problem. Should a patient need a larger dose his

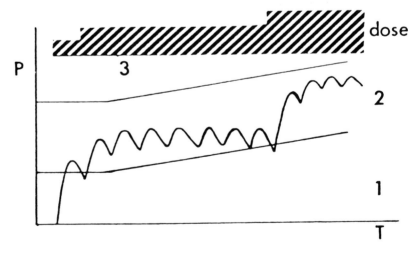

Figure 3 The effects of tolerance. Symbols: P = plasma drug concentration; T = time; 1 = no effect; 2 = useful effect; 3 = toxicity (Adapted from Vere[20])

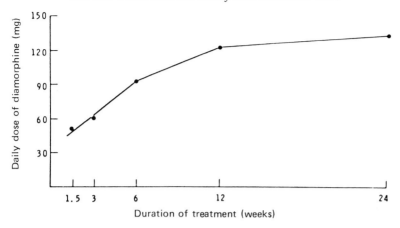

Figure 4 Change in daily dose of diamorphine with duration of treatment. 418 patients admitted consecutively with advanced cancer were grouped according to survival following the start of treatment with diamorphine; group median final daily dose of diamorphine is shown plotted against group median duration of treatment (after Twycross).

effective zone has shifted and this is as true for respiratory depression and other side effects as for analgesia. Sequential increases in oral doses are usually in increments of 5 mg for doses of less than 20 mg, then to 30 mg, 45 mg and 60 mg and thereafter each increase is usually in the range of 20–30 mg. The maximum effective oral dose is ill-defined but in our practice doses higher than 90 mg are seldom needed. (see Figure 5). As Twycross has shown (Figure 4) tolerance seems to level off in most cases and usually ceases to operate after a few weeks[21]. In many of the reported studies[6, 19, 21-23] phenothiazines were routinely given with the oral narcotic elixir. The usual practice has been to dispense these separately and to keep the dose relatively stable while altering the narcotic. Only one drug change should be made at a time. Other adjuvant medication should also be added individually. A degree of polypharmacy is indicated for most of these patients but this must be carefully monitored and regularly reviewed.

ABSORPTION OF ORAL NARCOTICS

In spite of longterm effective use in various centres objections are still heard concerning the use of oral narcotics on the grounds of poor and unreliable absorption. Although we still await further studies on the pharmacokinetics of these drugs, on the basis of urinary excretion studies, Twycross, Fry and Wills[24] estimated that diamorphine is probably completely absorbed from the gastrointestinal tract and that morphine is some two-thirds absorbed. Wynne Aherne, Piall and Twycross[25] have now reported a further study in which assay of serum 'morphine equivalents' was by radioimmunoassay. Venous blood from 65 patients receiving diamorphine hydrochloride and 24 morphine sulphate showed a highly significant positive linear correlation between the dose administered and the serum concentration ($p < 0.001$) with respect to both drugs[25].

THE LAST HOURS

Many patients become somewhat drowsy and confused in their last days. Much of this is due to the progress of their disease but Mount suggests[5] and we have observed ourselves that some people require less narcotic at this time and they may become relatively oversedated. If careful and skilled observation is possible we may follow this by a downward titration of the narcotic dose. On the other hand, patients who develop terminal restlessness may have increased pain with decreased ability to convey this to others and here we may well have to increase both the narcotic and the phenothiazine. Some patients develop jerking or twitching movements and although they may not be aware of this their visitors will be disturbed. An injection of diazepam 5–10 mg p.r.n. should give control. Fluid may accumulate in the lungs during the last hours and give rise to the 'death rattle'. If we prepare for this comparatively common occurrence and prescribe ahead for injections of hyoscine (Scopolamine) 0.4–0.6 mg together with the opiate, an experienced ward sister who will detect the first signs will nearly always prevent this added distress to the family and to other patients.

Terminal confused restlessness must be controlled with adequate sedation, especially in home care. Chlorpromazine is usually the phenothiazine of choice at this stage but methotrimeprazine (Veractil, Nozinan) is held in reserve and it is rare for an adequate dose (25–50 mg) to be ineffective.

WHICH OPIATE?

Because for some time we had a clinical impression that diamorphine is the opiate drug of choice a series of studies were carried out at the hospice with this drug[23.26].

From this work Twycross reported a controlled cross-over trial between morphine and diamorphine and he showed that given regularly at individually optimized doses in an elixir with cocaine and a phenothiazine there was no clinically observable difference[27]. As diamorphine is not available in most countries this was an important finding. The hospice changed its practice in 1977 and morphine is prescribed for all oral narcotic medication (i.e. for two thirds of doses given). Only a minority of patients receive large doses (Figure 5). Because of its greater

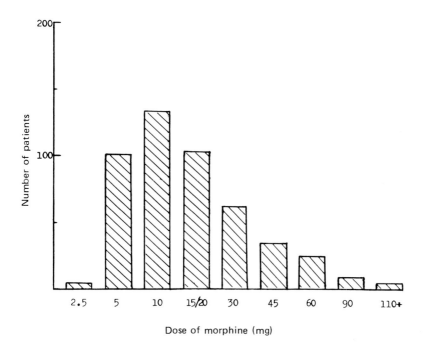

Dose of morphine (mg)

Figure 5 Oral morphine (1978) – maximum individual dose

solubility, diamorphine is retained for subcutaneous and intramuscular injections. This is monitored by the senior ward staff, at the appropriate time. The dose is scaled down in the ratio, oral morphine to injected diamorphine, 3:1 or oral to injected morphine, 2:1. At this stage chlorpromazine usually replaces prochlorperazine. The number of patients needing the larger doses and therefore larger volume is small and morphine would be an acceptable alternative for all but a small minority.

Experience suggests that when regularly administered oral morphine is used as the narcotic therapy of choice in this setting there will only infrequently be the need to broaden the armamentarium to include other agents. The only other strong analgesics likely to be prescribed in St. Christoper's are phenazocine and dextromoramide. Phenazocine (Narphen) is given when a patient dislikes the morphine elixir or prefers a tablet (5 mg are equivalent to 25 mg morphine). Dextromoramide (Palfium) is short-acting and is sometimes used for the rapid relief of an exacerbation of pain (5 mg equivalent to 15 mg morphine). Methadone is rarely prescribed. There is no problem of cumulation with morphine or diamorphine but the fate and excretion of methadone is more complex. Although it has been widely used with ambulant and fitter groups of patients, life-threatening cumulation may occur among the frail and elderly. Hospice patients treated with methadone showed a shorter survival than those given equi-effective doses of diamorphine or morphine[28].

THE BROMPTON MIXTURE

Mixtures under this and other titles and containing different amounts of one or more narcotic drugs are still widely used. Frequently hospital staff do not know what their own mixture contains and how little discrimination they may be using. Twycross studied the effect of cocaine in the St. Christopher's diamorphine mixture among 45 patients who completed a within patient comparison. Although patients crossing from no-cocaine to with-cocaine felt slightly more alert while receiving cocaine and females felt stronger, its cessation after 2 weeks did not appear to result in decreased alertness or a feeling of increased weakness[29]. This finding was later confirmed by Melzack, who compared a formula containing alcohol and cocaine to a simple aqueous solution of morphine in a double blind, crossover trial. There was no significant difference in mean morphine dose used, effectiveness of pain control attained or incidence of side effects encountered[30]. We may conclude that morphine in water or chloroform water, the traditional English vehicle for mixtures, is as effective as the previously popular mixtures and that the latter should be discontinued in view of confusion concerning the strength of the narcotic dose and the minimal effect and shortage of cocaine.

A solution is to be preferred in most cases because the dose can be titrated accurately to the patient's need and may be increased without enlarging the volume taken. A patient whose dose for pain control progresses from one to three or four tablets is reminded on each drug round of that increase. There are likely to be other tablets to swallow and this can be a burden in itself.

Alcohol was omitted from the St. Christopher's mixture without a controlled trial but drinks have always been given as part of the hospitality of the hospice. Offered in suitable glasses as a pre-supper drink and freely available if brought in by families and friends it enhances the normal social interchange for the patients in a way open to no other tranquillizer. Like other diversions, it may act as a potent relief of all forms of pain.

No one drug and no routine method is the whole answer to the control of terminal pain. Regular giving is not a panacea, it is a pattern into which other treatments and a general approach should be integrated.

Success in pain control is easier to achieve when realistic goals are set. A patient needing opiates for pain relief should usually be sleeping well within the first day or two. It is possible, especially with bone pain, that pain on movement may be more difficult to abolish and with a few patients this may never be fully achieved. However, once nights are good and rest during the day is pain-free, most of these patients will accept some change in their level of activity. Other reasons for continued distress are discussed below.

MENTAL PAIN

The patient's feelings or his insight into what is happening may well be his main problems and greatly exacerbate his total pain and undermine his capacity to cope with increasing weakness. Any illness causes anxiety and one that becomes more serious in spite of a variety of treatments until it is patently life-threatening will engender many fears. Patients tend to be left alone with these fears and only receive reassurance which they suspect is false or which has no relation to the anxiety they are facing. Mental suffering is likely to be enhanced by any physical distress and the doctor can do much to relieve the former whilst the other is being tackled. Competent symptom control brings support at a deep level and demands time with the patient and the close contact often denied at this stage. Isolation adds to the feeling of failure and the obscure sense of guilt suffered by many dying patients.

Studies of life changes have identified two main reactions occurring whenever a person is faced with the need to abandon one set of assumptions about his world and to adopt another[31]. On the one hand there is fear, apprehension and attempts to ward off the truth whilst on the other there is grief, mourning and a tendency to move towards the new situation. A dying patient needs time to work his way through and will be hindered by an ambiguous situation full of mismatched signals and deceptions. Fears are not removed by the pretence that they are without cause. Not everyone wishes to look at facts directly and it would be wrong to suggest a general rule that would mean assaulting people with truths which they were not ready to handle. However, anxiety does become less threatening when it has been expressed and some explanation given, even one that is hard to accept. In this way, the patient faces something he can worry through and not a vague shadow of disaster impossible to encompass in thought.

Hinton studied 80 patients dying in four different settings, two where the policy was to avoid any discussion of unpalatable truth and two which encouraged attempts to communicate more honestly. The latter group was less anxious and depressed and welcomed the greater openness[32]. Although no general principle can tell us what we must do to help the individual patient, it can give us guidelines and encouragement not to take automatically the easy (for us) way of evasion. When acknowledged fears are unrealistic we can provide reassurance and when they are realistic we can endeavour to help the patient face impending losses and express the grief that is indeed appropriate. When we have been honest in the past our reassurances that pain will not be allowed to escape control and that death itself will be peaceful are more likely to be accepted.

Fears of parting, of what will happen to dependents, of pain and of failing to cope are all realistic fears, common among dying patients[33]. Although the complexity of the problems faced by some are daunting it need not make us feel hopeless. Dying is not a psychiatric illness and does not usually call for specialized skills in counselling. Those who distance themselves feeling they can bring nothing but a lack of comprehension do not realize that it is their attempt to understand and not success in doing so that eases the patient's loneliness. The only visitor who helped the dying Ivan Ilych was the peasant boy who came with simple good will[34].

Nurses are closer to their patients than most doctors and are likely to hear more of a patient's questions and fears. Team consultations are essential if we are to reach helpful understanding. The social worker can listen in a unique way, for she is not involved with therapy and has been trained to act as the recipient of unacceptable feelings and projected angers; these are better expressed than buried only to appear in different guise. Contact with physiotherapists offers more than the pleasure of assisted movement or even the joy of tackling the stairs again, with the consequent reward of the weekend home. It is well known that the interested ward orderly may know more than anyone of matters which a patient does not feel able to share with the professionals who surround him. We must not forget that boredom may be a major component of mental pain and a good gossip, like other distractions is often the best way to relieve it.

If we are prepared to talk frankly with a patient, it does not mean that this will necessarily happen but there is now a new freedom in which we can wait for clues from each patient, seeing them as people from whom we expect intelligence, courage and individual decisions.

Truth is likely to emerge gradually and those who have listened constantly to dying patients have seen many progress into realization of their situation and come to terms with it. A well known system has been described by Ross[35], who details a development through stages of denial and isolation, anger or protest, bargaining and depression into a final acceptance. She has emphasized that not all will follow this course clearly but her work seems to have encouraged others with less sensitivity to impose this structure upon their patients to the detriment of true listening and individual response. People are as individual in their dying as they are in their living. Persistent cancer follows an irregular and unpredictable course and the patient may face a number of disappointments, each one of which must be grieved before the person is ready to move on[33]. We need constantly to be alert to changes in our patient's situation and his reaction to it.

The psychotropic drugs may help in bringing the burden of his illness within a particular patient's compass and they are widely used. Their prescription as adjuvants to analgesics has been discussed above. The narcotic group of drugs are themselves powerful tranquillizers and some of their effectiveness stems from this fact. Most dying patients are likely to have a drug of the phenothiazine group prescribed but little definitive work has been carried out in this area. The tricyclic group of drugs are also used empirically, though less frequently by most workers in this field. At times they are extremely useful but many patients do not appear to require them. In St. Christopher's Hospice 16% of all patients are prescribed a drug of the tricyclic group but this figure rises to 39% for those who remain as patients for more than three months[26]. A patient with an endogenous or severe reactive depression stands out in a ward of dying patients as does to a lesser extent one who has developed a chronic pain syndrome. These problems do not arise with most patients who die of malignant disease but are an occasional challenge that may need specialist advice.

Most people will finally accept the approach of death as they accept other forms of loss, although the faint hope of an unexpected recovery or remission is common until near the end and not to be discouraged. Hope in different forms can exist all through illness, gradually changing its content. This grows out of the realistic facing of problems and helps the patient to accept the responsibility of living the life that remains to him.

SOCIAL PAIN

When an illness has a foreseeable end most families will come to grips with the situation and will wish to look after a dying relative at home as long as possible. Although the trend is for a higher proportion of cancer deaths to occur in hospital, prolongation of life by the newer treatments frequently means that much of this extra time is spent at home. Only a minority will require heavy nursing for any length of time but there may be a prolonged period of emotional strain for patient and family alike. If they can be helped to handle this it may be an important time for them all for it enables the survivors to prepare for parting and to make some restitution for the failures of the past. Old tensions may become acute but even at this stage, often because it *is* the final stage, reconciliation is not uncommon and many people make this a remarkably fruitful time. The dependence of the sick person strengthens attachment and many people cope heroically with the heavy burdens of care. Others cannot handle the emotions involved and some families have such complicated problems that the help of a caseworker may be essential. The hospice movement in the USA is developing mainly in the home care setting and here the work of the doctor and the social worker is supplemented by experienced nurses and specially trained volunteers, often with a professional background.

It is essential that someone should not only make available additional help but also inform the family beforehand that this is possible. Financial burdens are often heavy especially for those who have prolonged time off work but the patient should be included in all discussions and plans as he should be involved as far as possible in normal family life. The two reactions to impending changes in life noted above will operate within all members of the family. As they try to ward off threatening changes and at the same time find themselves making an attempt to face and handle them it is all too easy for different members to get badly out of step with each other and with the patient. The patient who is kept in the dark about family finances and various practical matters will have the added burden of fancying he has hurt or offended the others because of the barriers thus erected.

There is a tradition in this country of families withholding truth from the sick relative. One can understand the strong desire to keep all worries from the patient, yet this protectiveness frequently leads to crippling tensions and it is sad since the patient is likely to come to know the truth by other means. To keep an unshared secret from an intimate inevitably impairs communication and can add greatly to the sum of the patient's distress. 'The successful open sharing of their stress which comes about spontaneously in some marital relationships has a quality which leads one to hope that more could be helped by a similar achievement'[36]. Admission to a hospice may greatly ease family anxiety. Thirty-four patients who had died in St. Christopher's were matched with 34 who had died in general hospitals in the area. One major difference was the amount of anxiety the spouses reported before and after admission. Spouses describing their anxiety as very great before and after admission changed in the St. Christopher's setting from 85% to 22% and in the other hospital settings from 57% to 36%.

The New Haven Hospice team, assessing their work among patients and families in their own homes, found a similar change and that the main significant differences from a matched group occurred among the families rather than among the patients themselves[37]. Home care is the choice of most people whenever this can be made possible by good symptom control and general support and over 70% of the New Haven patients now die in their own homes. The Macmillan Home Care Service attached to St. Joseph's Hospice, Hackney, report that 55% of their patients are enabled to die at home. These two teams are both involved in much of the nursing and the prescribing. The St. Christopher's Home Care Team, established in 1969, works alongside the community doctors and services as a consultative support group and has a much lower figure of home deaths although the median final stay in the hospice is only half that of a group of patients without hospice support[38].

Admission may bring comfort for the patient and reduction of anxiety for the family which must not be bought at the cost of feelings of guilt.

The family must be reassured that they have done what they could and that professional help is now needed on a full-time basis. The ward staff must not take over care in such a way as to exclude the family, who can contribute greatly to his security and peace by their mere presence and this should be made possible and explicit. Every member of staff should be able to give some recognition, even though brief, to the family that is maintaining its last watch with a dying member.

The long pain of the family's bereavement is a part of terminal pain. They will begin to grieve their imminent parting during the illness but the real letting go and approach to the new situation will rarely happen before the patient dies. The final watch and the witnessing of a peaceful death may be very important for some families whilst others cannot remain by the bedside. It may not be possible or advisable and care must be taken to protect them from feelings of guilt and responsibility at this time. Ward staff are all too familiar with the desolation of the final moment of parting and the empty numbness that follows it but do not always appreciate how greatly their supporting presence can ease even this.

Some families may ask for sedatives. This is probably mistaken. Grief needs to be expressed at this point and drugs may inhibit this natural and eventually healing reaction. There is no ground for prescribing tranquillizers or anti-depressants to the bereaved as a routine. Parkes believes that such drugs should be reserved for the potentially suicidal and for those who, despite all efforts to help, remain in a state of chronic agitation or depression[33]. A mild hypnotic may be needed for those whose sleep is continually disturbed.

The bereaved family comes slowly to full realization of what has happened and after often intense inner struggle and dejection is eventually ready to build a new life. This may take many months and is felt like a sort of illness which is finally healed. Abnormal, unresolved grief needs skilled help.

The whole process of bereavement is not often seen by clinicians other than family doctors but we should all accept two responsibilities. Firstly, to see that others are alert to identifying and helping those who are especially at risk in their loss and secondly, to do all that is possible to ease the memories of those who live on.

Most dying people show remarkable endurance and those who spend their time close to them find that this helps to reduce their own fears of death. The dying have a good heritage to leave which is not always recognized nor received. Parkes writes of his admiration for many of the people who have shared their grief with him and finds that counselling the bereaved makes it easier to recognize bereavement as an acceptable part of life[33].

SPIRITUAL PAIN

Not many people are likely to express the suffering of their doubts and griefs in religious terms. Nevertheless, feelings of failure, regret and meaninglessness which may be the deepest element in the 'total pain' are spiritual needs. Liaison with a priest or minister of the patient's own choice may then be important. The ward sister is often the person with whom the hospital chaplain has the most to do but contact with the doctor may be essential. Consultation is most effective when it is personal, informal and continuing. It would be unwarranted intrusion to suggest such a contact when there is no understanding or willingness on the part of the patient but in spite of the gap that seems to exist between minister or priest and people we will often be surprised how welcome such a visit can be.

Our regard for our patient will never allow us to impose upon him but unspoken confidence and belief may create a climate in which the patient may find his own key and reach out to what he sees as valuable and true.

STAFF PAIN

The supporters themselves frequently need supporting, especially during their first weeks in terminal care. Its demands cause pain and bewilderment at times to all in this field and the closer the staff are to the weakness of the patients and the grief of the families the more they too will suffer the pangs of bereavement. Many will find they are suffering the process of numbness and exhaustion, protest, anger and depression and will need to share this if they are to find their way through. The resilience of those who continue to work in this field is won by a full understanding of what is happening and not by a retreat behind a technique.

Group meetings are likely to be needed as well as the regular ward discussions concerned with distressing or difficult patients and families. Much support will be informal and come from the peer group of the one who is finding that stress has become too great. Friends and interests

completely outside the work are essential as is the awareness and sup
port of senior staff, for each must find an outlet and a way of expressing
and working through this pain.

Efficiency is always comforting. The giving of effective relief to all types
of pain makes this an extremely rewarding field. Nevertheless, if we are
to remain for long near the suffering of dependence and parting
we need to develop a basic philosophy and search, often painfully, for
meaning in even the most adverse situations. We have to gain enough
confidence in what we are doing and enough freedom from our anxieties
to listen to another's distress. In this coming together we may see something of the achievements that relief of terminal pain can make possible.

Our competence in the control of terminal pain is there to give our patients and their families freedom to make the best use of the time that
remains to them.

References

1 Smithers, D. W. (1960). *A Clinical Prospect of the Cancer Problem.* (Edinburgh: Livingstone)
2 Parkes, C. M. (1978). Home or hospital? Patterns of care for the terminally ill cancer patient as seen by surviving spouses. *J. R. Coll. Gen. Practitioners*, **28**, 19
3 Woodbine, G. (1977). The Care of Patients Dying From Cancer, A Cross-Sectional Study. *MSc Thesis*, University of Southampton
4 Hunt, J. M., Stollar, T. D., Littlejohns, D. W., Twycross, R. G. and Vere, D. W. (1977). Patients with protracted pain: A survey conducted at the London Hospital, *J. Med Ethics*, **3**, 61
5 Mount, B. M. (1979). Narcotic Analgesics. Presented at the *International Seminar on Continuing Care of Terminal Cancer Patients*, October 19–20, Milan
6 Melzack, R., Ofiesh, J. G. and Mount, B. M. (1976). The Brompton mixture: effects on pain in cancer patients. *Canad. Med. Assoc. J.*, **115**, 125
7 Evans, R. J. (1971). Experiences in a pain clinic. *Mod. Med. Canada*
8 Wall, P. D. (1979). On the relation of injury to pain. The John J. Bonica Lecture. *Pain*, **6**, 253
9 Beecher, H. K. (1960). *Quantitative Effect of Drugs, (Harvard University)* (London and New York: Oxford University Press)
10 Calman, K. C., Murdoch, J. C. (1974). What does the general practitioner want to know about the cancer patient? *Lancet*, **2**, 770
11 Bates, T. D. (1978). Radiotherapy in terminal care. In Saunders, Cicely, M. (ed.) *The Management of Terminal Disease* (London: Edward Arnold)
12 Clarke, I. M. C. (1980). Personal communication
13 Baines, M. (1977). *Drug Control of Common Symptoms* World Medicine Publication
14 Baines, M. (1978). Control of other symptoms. In Saunders, Cicely, M. (ed.) *The Management of Terminal Disease.* (London: Edward Arnold)
15 Mount, B. M. (1978). Palliative care of the terminally ill. Presented at the *Annual Meeting of The Royal College of Physicians and Surgeons of Canada*, January 27, Vancouver

16 Falkson, G. (1979). Personal communication

17 Bonica, J. J. (1979). Cancer Pain: Importance of the Problem. In Bonica, J. J. and Ventafridda, V. (eds.) *Advances in Pain Research and Therapy* Vol 2, pp. 1–12. (New York: Raven Press)

18 Morris, J. C. (1959). The management of cases in the terminal stages of malignant disease. *St. Mary's Hospital Gazette*, **65,** 4

19 Saunders, C. M. (1967). *The Management of Terminal Illness.* (London: Hospital Medicine Publications)

20 Vere, D. W. (1978). *Topics in Therapeutics*, 4. (London: Pitman)

21 Twycross, R. G. (1978). Relief of pain. In Saunders, Cicely, M. (ed.) *The Management of Terminal Disease.* (London: Edward Arnold)

22 Mount, B. M., Ajemian, I. and Scott, J. F. (1976). Use of the Brompton mixture in treating the chronic pain of malignant disease, *Canad. Med. J.*, **115,** 122

23 Twycross, R. G. (1974). Clinical experience with diamorphine in advanced malignant disease, *Int. J. Clin. Pharmacol.*, **9,** 184

24 Twycross, R. G., Fry, D. E. and Wills, P. D. (1974). *Br. J. Clin. Pharmacol.*, **1,** 491

25 Wynne Aherne, G., Piall, E. and Twycross, R. G. (1979). Serum morphine concentration after oral administration of diamorphine hydrochloride and morphine sulphate. *Br. J. Clin. Pharmacol.*, **8,** 577

26 Twycross, R. G. and Wald, S. J. (1976). Longterm use of diamorphine in advanced cancer. In Bonica J. J. and Albe-Fessard, D. (eds.) *Advances in Pain Research and Therapy*, Vol. 1. (New York: Raven Press)

27 Twycross, R. G. (1977). Choice of strong analgesic in terminal cancer: diamorphine or morphine? *J. Int. Assoc. Stud. Pain*, **3,** 2

28 Twycross, R. G. (1976). Studies on the use of diamorphine in advanced malignant disease. *DM Thesis*, University of Oxford

29 Twycross, R. G. (1979). Effect of cocaine in the Brompton cocktail. In Bonica, J. J. and Albe-Fessard, D. (eds.) *Advances in Pain Research and Therapy*, Vol. 3. (New York: Raven Press)

30 Melzack, R., Mount, B. M. and Gordon, J. M. (1979). The Brompton mixture versus morphine solution given orally: effects on pain. *Canad. Med. J.*, **120,** 435

31 Parkes, C. M. (1973). Attachment and autonomy at the end of life. In R. Gosling (ed.) *Support, Innovation and Autonomy*, (London: Tavistock)

32 Hinton, J. (1979). Comparison of places and policies for terminal care. *Lancet*, **1,** 29

33 Parkes, C. M. (1978). Psychological aspects. In Saunders Cicely, M. (ed.) *The Management of Terminal Disease.* (London: Edward Arnold)

34 Tolstoy, L. (1886). *War and Peace.* (London: Oxford University Press)

35 Ross, E. K. (1970). *On Death and Dying.* (London: Tavistock)

36 Hinton, J. (1970). Communication between husband and wife in terminal cancer. Presented at the *Second International Conference on Social Science and Medicine*, 7–11 September, Aberdeen

37 Lack, S. A. and Buckingham, R. W. (1978). *First American Hospice: Three Years of Home Care.* (New Haven, Connecticut: Hospice Inc.)

38 Parkes, C. M. (1980). Evaluation of an advisory domiciliary service for terminal care. (In press)

Index

morphine
  analgesic effect mechanism   23
  clearance   91
  epidural   65
  long acting   93
  oral in terminal care   230–2
  postoperative and persistent pain   22
  steric arrangement   90
  subarachnoid   65
moxibustion   183
multiple myeloma, pain management   208
myofascial pain   172, 175
  fibrositic   175

naftidofuryl   108
nalbuphine   95
naloxone   89, 95, 96
naltrexone   89
naproxen   99
narcotic analgesics   88–96, 100
  mode of action   88, 89
  oral   228–30
    absorption   229, 230
  routes in cancer   93
  tolerance   228, 229
needle techniques   69
nefopam   65, 99
nerve block
  in chronic pain relief   111–31
  coeliac plexus   78, 124, 125, 155
  complications   127–9
  extradural   116, 117
  and local anaesthesia   111
  lumbar sympathetic block   66, 76, 78
  non-neurolytic   129–31
  peripheral   124–9
    lumbar sympathectomy   66, 76, 78,
      125, 126
    peripheral somatic blocks   126, 127
    post-traumatic sympathetic dystrophy
      126
  pituitary ablation   120–2
  subarachnoid   114–16, 128
    alcohol rhizotomy   114
    techniques   115, 116
  subdural   117–19, 128
    intrathecal saline   117–19
    technique   119
  trigeminal neurolysis   122–4
    complications   123
    technique   122

neuralgia *see also* trigeminal neuralgia
  glossopharyngeal   144
  nervus intermedius   145
  occipital   147
  post cholecystectomy   161
  postherpetic   10, 103, 154
  vagal   144
neurectomy, peripheral   142
neuritis   113
neurology   1–29
neurolytic agents
  complications   127–9
  hazards   113
neurolytic solutions   85
neurosurgery *see also* rhizotomy
  analgesia   136
  cingulumotomy   166
  cerebral targets   164–6
  CNS stimulation   162, 163
  cordotomy   74, 76, 121, 152–5, 158, 159
    bilateral   159
    complications   153
    follow up   158, 159
  craniofacial pain   138–47
  facial pain   46
  mesencephalotomy   164
  myelotomy   153, 156, 157
  orbitofrontal leucotomy   17
  in pain relief   135–66
  stereotactic   152, 153
  stereotactic thalamotomy   17, 158
  sympathectomy   161, 162
  thalamotomy   164–6
    technique   165
  tractotomy   160
  trigeminal neuralgia   138–43
  trunk and pelvic pain   147–57
nociceptive receptors
  activation   6, 8
  interstitial   4, 5
  and irritation   6, 8
  perivascular   5
  plexiform   5
nociceptive relays, brainstem   12, 13
nociceptive stimulation
  polysynaptic connections   7, 8
  spinal reflexogenic effects   8
nociceptive stimulus   2
nociceptive system
  central projections   11–19
    central   11, 12